CONTEMPORARY COMMUNITY HEALTH SERIES

Titles in the Series

CHILDREN IN JEOPARDY
A Study of Abused Minors and Their Families
Elizabeth Elmer

HOME TREATMENT
Spearhead of Community Psychiatry
Leonard Weiner, Alvin Becker, Tobias T. Friedman

EDUCATION AND MANPOWER
FOR COMMUNITY HEALTH
Hilary G. Fry, with William P. Shepard and Ray H. Elling

MIGRANTS AND MALARIA IN AFRICA
R. Mansell Prothero

DENTISTS, PATIENTS, AND AUXILIARIES
Margaret Cussler and Evelyn W. Gordon

ANATOMY OF A COORDINATING COUNCIL
Implications for Planning
Basil J. F. Mott

BRITISH PRIVATE MEDICAL PRACTICE
AND THE NATIONAL HEALTH SERVICE
Samuel Mencher

British Private Medical Practice

AND THE NATIONAL HEALTH SERVICE

British
Private Medical Practice

AND THE
NATIONAL HEALTH SERVICE

by

SAMUEL ⌐MENCHER

University of Pittsburgh Press

Library of Congress Catalog Card Number 68–21629

Copyright © 1968, University of Pittsburgh Press

Manufactured in the United States of America

Contents

Foreword   ix

Preface   xi

Acknowledgments   xv

1 Private Practice: An Overview   1

2 Private Health Insurances   14

3 The Patient and Private Practice   30

4 Issues for Private Practice   37

5 Private Practice: The Doctors' Dilemma   68

6 The Future for Private Practice   98

Notes   105

Index   121

Foreword

SAMUEL Mencher, scholar, teacher, and friend, died suddenly on March 10, 1967. All who are concerned with the social welfare problems of modern society experienced a profound sense of loss at his untimely death. His contribution in furthering our understanding of the dilemmas of social policy in the United States was a remarkable one. In his teaching, his research, and his writing he combined a painstaking respect for the facts with a deep appreciation of the play of historical forces in shaping and molding policies for the relief of poverty, the provision of medical care, and the development of welfare systems in general.

Few American scholars, working in these fields, have so well understood simultaneously the social policy problems of their own society and of British society. He often returned, in much that he wrote, to the theme of the common origins of welfare in the old Elizabethan Poor Law, and continued to puzzle about the divergent paths followed by social legislation in the two countries since the eighteenth century.

Sam visited Britain as often as he could and spent one sabbatical year in 1953–54 at the London School of Economics and Political Science for his doctoral thesis in child welfare services, and one year in 1965–66 at Manchester University. In the early 1960's, intellectually involved as he was in the American debate on medical care, he became more interested in the role of government in the field of health. He thus set out, on his arrival in Manchester, to study the survival in Britain of private practice since the introduction of the National Health Service in 1948.

What was—and is—its future? What are the problems, professional and administrative, of two standards of practice for the general practitioner? What conflicts have beset the medical profession in emphasizing the role of "independent contractor" and in aiming to provide for all their patients, public and private, the best possible medical care which the total resources of modern medicine can now make available? These and allied questions formed the starting-point of this study of private practice in Britain, which was completed only a few weeks before Sam died.

On behalf of all his friends and colleagues in the United States and Britain I am glad to have had this opportunity to pay tribute to the contribution that Samuel Mencher made to human welfare.

Richard M. Titmuss
August 1967

Preface

THE transition of the British health professions and services into a highly complex public system has been a phenomenon of intriguing interest to the social scientist. Although other fields of service have been transferred and continue to be transferred from the private to the public sphere, they have not been the source of comparable conflict. Any major shift of function arouses, even if only ritualistically, the parading of ideological differences, but in most bureaucratically organized services change of sponsorship has only minor consequences for those directly engaged in providing the service. For teachers, engineers, social workers, and even those elements of the health professions, such as nurses and research and laboratory workers who are members of an organized structure of service, there has always been a contract of employment and a recognition that effective professional performance depended on organizational supports. In these as well as in other professions, there may be those who practice individually or privately but, unlike the medical profession where there are many directly employed on the staffs of health institutions, these professions have not maintained an image or ideal of professional performance identified with independent practice.

Thus, the continuance of private medical service in Britain some twenty years after the National Health Service Act highlights the'strains and stresses peculiar to the practice of medicine during the first generation of the Health Service. In addition, the nature, the extent, and the growth or decline of private practice are crude, yet important indicators of public response. Finally, although the coexistence of public and private medicine in Britain has unique cultural features, it brings to the fore many of the fundamental issues of health and social policy generally. Broadly speaking, what are the consequences for society and effective provision of health of the presence of two approaches to health care? What is the nature of the interaction between the two approaches and its significance for the performance of each? For, in the last analysis, the British experience indicates that the role of private medicine can only be understood in the context of the broad public provision of health care.

Apart from a brief reminder of the situation prior to 1948, this study has concentrated on appraising the functioning of private medicine since the National Health Service Act. So much scholarly attention has already been given to the crucial years of the formulation of the plan and the negotiations between the medical profession and the government that a firm foundation for contemporary analysis may be assumed.[1] However, starting with the terms of the agreement reached, what has been the continuing history of accommodation between the practice of private medicine and the structure established in 1948? Specifically, attention will be given to trends in the amount and types of private medicine, the role of the private health insurances, the issues of conflict between private medicine and public policy, the attitude of the public, and the complex position of the medical profession.

In addition to available published materials, this study is based upon one year of research in England during which the author had the opportunity of interviewing and discussing the issues with, among others, the leadership of the professional medical associations, the executives of the health insurance societies, and a small but selected sample of general practitioners and consultants engaged in private practice. Except where strictly factual material has been involved, interviews with the members of the medical profession have been used to suggest hypotheses rather than incorporated as conclusive data. While not representative in the strictly scientific sense of the term, these interviews provided invaluable insights to supplement the interpretation of other data.

S. M.

Acknowledgments

I WISH to express appreciation for the interest and cooperation of the many persons related to the health services who were hospitable and helpful during my stay in England. The staff of the Ministry of Health, the B.M.A., the voluntary health insurances, and other organizations concerned with the provision of health care were most cooperative. Max Ward of the Western Provident Association was particularly helpful in making data available on the private insurances as were John H. Dyter of the Hospital Service Plan and E. D. Roberts of B.U.P.A. Miss Dora Livock provided most useful historical material on the development of the private insurances.

At the University of Manchester Mr. A. R. Anscombe, Dean of Clinical Studies, and Professor T. E. Chester and Mr. Gordon Forsyth of the Department of Social Administration, were most cooperative in suggesting sources and discussing the study. Professor Titmuss and Professor Abel-Smith of the London School of Economics and Political Science provided much friendly advice. The investigation was supported in part by a Public Health Service Fellowship from the National Institute of Health of the U.S. Department of Health, Education and Welfare.

British Private Medical Practice

AND THE NATIONAL HEALTH SERVICE

CHAPTER 1

Private Practice: An Overview

THE creation of the National Health Service, like other major instruments of social policy, symbolized a new era of social provision. Although it crystalized radical reforms of earlier institutions, it represented more a hastening of processes already underway than a repudiation of the past. The Appointed Day in 1948 when the Service began was neither the beginning of public medicine nor the end of private practice. Both systems had existed before the Act and continued after its operation. The Act made significant changes in the nature of each and their relationship to each other, but the Service was "conditioned" by its inheritance of the attitudes and culture of previous medical practice.[1]

Prior to 1948, some 24 million persons or almost half the population of Great Britain were covered by the National Health Insurance Scheme established in 1912.[2] This scheme provided general practitioner care, drugs, and a limited amount of surgical and medical appliances without charge for insured persons. Only employed persons with wages of less than £420 per year were provided for, and beneficiaries did not include wives, children, and other dependents of insured persons. These services were supplemented by the out-patients' departments of the voluntary hospitals which further reduced the numbers wholly dependent on private medical care. Thus, private practice probably catered to somewhat less than half the population.[3]

As under the present scheme, doctors elected voluntarily to participate. About two-thirds of all doctors served National Health Insurance patients, and it has been estimated that about one-third of the average doctor's income came from the annual capitation fees of the scheme.[4] The proportion of doctors and the amount of their income from the scheme varied from area to area. In highly industrialized regions, doctors' practices were much more dependent on Health Insurance patients than in wealthy or rural areas. By 1948, there were already many doctors whose practices closely resembled the type of practice prevalent after the National Health Service Act. Not only had they large panel practices; they had also lengthy experience with the supervisory and regulatory controls established by the state.[5] On the other hand, there were large numbers of doctors who had minimal contact with the public scheme. These differences help to account in some measure for differences in attitudes and responses of doctors after 1948.

As distinct from the present scheme, the earlier Act only provided limited benefits to those covered. There was, for example, no provision for hospital care, nursing after-care, X-ray diagnosis and treatment, physiotherapy, or orthopedic appliances or artificial limbs.[6] Some of the Approved Societies which administered the scheme gave additional benefits, but these were extremely irregular and, at best, applied only to optical and dental needs.[7] To guard against the costs of hospital care many people joined hospital contributory schemes, organized by voluntary societies. These undertook to meet some of the costs of hospitalization, and by 1947 the British Hospitals Contributory Schemes Association reported a total of ten and one-half million members with benefits also extending to their dependents.[8]

The hospital contributory schemes were originally organized as charitable collections for the voluntary hospitals but gradually became hospital insurance funds for low-income groups. In principle, the schemes insisted on their role as supporters of the voluntary hospital system, but in practice and eventually even in policy they recognized as among their purposes:

> To enable wage-earners and others (with limited incomes) . . . to obtain Hospital privileges for themselves and their dependents by means of an organised system of regular contributors, in return for which the contributors . . . will be relieved from Hospital charges when receiving Hospital treatment.[9]

By the 1940's, contributory associations were providing about 50 per cent of the total income of voluntary hospitals.

The contributory schemes limited their membership to persons of low income; in 1938, for example, the maximum weekly income for membership was between four and five pounds.[10] Although there was pressure for the schemes to meet the full cost of care, it was assumed that they would only make partial payment.[11] In effect, the schemes guaranteed the hospitals some amount of payment for patients for whom they might otherwise have had to provide all or almost all of their service free.

From the patient's point of view, membership freed him from the unpleasantness and indignities of income inquiries normally conducted when charitable hospital care was sought. With this in mind, the hospitals and the associations were particularly chary of extending membership to those who might be able to pay privately for their treatment.[12]

However, even for those who, it was assumed, could pay privately the cost of hospital care was a heavy burden. Such contributory schemes as the large Hospital Savings Association of London began to extend their coverage to somewhat higher income levels. A new group of societies, the provident societies, were organized to meet the needs of the middle class, and by the end of the 1930's, all restrictions on income were removed for membership. Within certain income limits, total costs would be met; above these limits, fixed payments would be made toward the cost arranged by private agreement of the patient and the hospital staff.[13]

In addition to the rising charges for hospital beds themselves, the increasing cost of care for the more well-to-do was affected by the fees of the consultants and specialists on the hospital staff. Originating as charitable institutions, the hospitals had made no charge for medical services. But there was a gradual development of pay beds in the twentieth century, and this trend became greatly accelerated during the thirties. These beds would provide more luxurious accommodation for those who could afford to pay both the extra maintenance charges for the beds and the private fees of the consultants and specialists in attendance. These fees gradually became a more important part of the consultants' incomes as, it was alleged, consultant income had been reduced by the use of the hospital for services which the consultant had previously provided privately.[14] The principle of the paid consultant was also evolving in still another direction with some of the municipal hospitals engaging consultants on a part or whole sessional salary.[15] Thus, consultants, who had earlier served the hospitals on a gratuitous basis and gained their income largely from private practice outside the hospitals, came to view the hospital as their chief source of income.

The largest proportion of hospital facilities was administered by the local authorities. They had inherited the old Poor Law hospitals and institutions and had been given the power, in 1930, to expand general hospital facilities. Like the voluntary hospitals, these cared for both paying and charitable cases, and the contributory insurance schemes were used to pay for hospital maintenance by members receiving treatment in local authority hospitals. Under the Poor Law, hospital medical staff had been employed on a full- or part-time salaried basis. This practice was continued in the public general hospitals, but did not prove an attractive method for recruiting and staffing medical personnel. When the public hospitals turned to employing part-time consultants, these consultants began to supplement their salaries with income from fees paid by patients in private beds.[16]

The Poor Law, in addition to its in-patient responsibilities, provided general practitioners services for the sick poor in their own homes. This, too, had been administered by part-time and full-time salaried doctors. Changes occurred also in this service when some of the authorities introduced the panel system whereby assistance recipients could use any doctor in the area who agreed to accept them. The British Medical Association was influential in having a capitation system of payment substituted for compensation based on fee-for-service.[17]

Thus, in general, the forms of public and private practice were established during several decades before the National Health Service and particularly in the period between the end of World War I and 1948. The general practitioner received his income from capitation payments for public patients and from the fees of private patients. Specialists and consultants, apart from private consultations, had private arrangements with paying hospital patients, and these payments might or might not be supplemented by a sessional salary from the hospital. Only the poorest received free treatment. The remainder of the population resorted to the contributory and provident schemes for meeting hospital costs. The latter also made provision as well for the payment of specialist services, and there was a general trend to expand the nature of the benefits under the schemes.

This structure of public and private practice continued after the National Health Service although there were major changes in the quality and distribution of medical services which diminished the sharp distinction between public and private medicine. As an eminent physician whose career has spanned both periods commented:

The division of mankind into private patients on the one hand and hospital or panel patients on the other was much more in evidence than it is today. The latter were often very decently and devotedly served by doctors in varying types of practice and by the consultants and residents of the hospitals . . . but in some cases the standards of working class General Practice were fairly appalling, and in hospital patients were expected to be grateful but undemanding; to be seen but not heard. There were some surgeons . . . who seemed to have no regard for patients' feelings. . . . Amongst the physicians, the frequent demands of private practice would make inroads into the time they spent in hospital work, all of which was of course unpaid.[18]

The National Health Service, as conceived by both the Conservative and Labour governments which preceded its enactment, was not to be the single and sole purveyor of medical care for the nation. Doctors and patients would have the right to remain outside the Service. As the White Paper of the Conservative government stated in 1944:

> If anyone prefers not to use it, or likes to make private arrangements outside the service, he must be at liberty to do so. Similarly, if any medical practitioner prefers not to take part in the new service, and to rely wholly on private work outside it, he also must be at liberty to do so.[19]

This principle was further delineated in the Labour government's paper of 1946 which, although its interpretation was to be the source of later controversy, provided that "all the service, or any part of it, is to be available to everyone in England and Wales."[20] In effect, a person might select to receive some of his medical care privately without losing his privilege to other elements of the public service.

A general practitioner might remain entirely in private practice or have a mixed practice of private patients and patients registered on his National Health Service panel. Apart from paying for the practitioner's service and drugs, the private patient would be eligible for all other treatment within and outside the hospital system. His physician, for example, whether wholly or partially in private practice, could provide or have provided for the private patient medical certificates, maternity care, specialist consultations, district nursing and home-help services, and all in- and outpatient hospital facilities.

A specialist or consultant, too, might choose to be entirely in private practice or might accept a part-time rather than whole-time contract with a regional hospital board. As a fully private consultant, his hospital practice would be limited to those hospital facilities outside of the National Health Service. A small group of clinics and hospitals, some sponsored by religious orders and other organizations, had not been incorporated in the national system. There were also private nursing homes which catered to the hospital needs of the more wealthy. The part-time National Health Service consultant might also use these facilities, but he had the advantage as well of specially designated private beds in the National Health Service hospitals on whose staff he served. He could, as well, maintain his own private consultation practice outside the hospital. Although the whole-time consultant cannot continue in private practice, he, like the general practitioner, may charge fees for services that are not covered by his responsibilities under the Act. Routine tests and examinations required by organizations, vaccinations for travel, and contraceptives prescribed on non-medical grounds, fall into this category.

These are, however, relatively minor sources of income from private practice. The most significant source of private income are the pay beds under Section 5 of the Act. Three basic types of hospital accommodation are provided under the National Health Service. All patients are eligible for free hospital and specialist services. Those desiring more privacy may receive such accommodation, under Section 4, for an extra charge fixed to cover part of the cost. Apart from occupying "amenity" beds they are similar in all other respects to the mass of National Health Service patients. A third class of patients are those who occupy private beds established for patients who are prepared to pay the full cost of treatment and accommodation. These are generally the patients of private consultants and specialists whose patients pay for their services in addition to the full hospital charges.

The amount of private practice or service to patients outside the National Health Service, although the source of some interest in Britain, has not been easy to measure. There is no accurate reporting of those engaged in private practice, the number of private patients, or the income from private practice as there is in the case of medical care under the National Health Service. The British Medical Association's list of private practitioners depends on self-reporting by doctors. General surveys of doctors and patients are influenced by the greater probability of failure to respond or unreliable responses among those outside the conventional field of public medicine. Even when this is not the case, the numbers involved are frequently so small and the variations among areas so great as to make questionable the suggested estimates from studies of medical practice.

A survey of general medical practice in 1964 indicated that almost one-third of the practitioners had no private patients, over three-quarters had less than twenty patients, and only 4 per cent had at least one hundred patients.[21] A study of a smaller sample of National Health Service doctors conducted in 1963 by the same researcher found that almost one-quarter of the general practitioners had no private practice and 14 per cent had 100 or more private patients.[22] However, the variations may be accounted for by the differences in the areas included in the study samples. Of the thirteen areas surveyed in the 1963 study, two accounted for half the doctors with private practices of 100 or more patients. In the 1964 study, differences among the areas sampled were less extreme, and it is likely that any general practitioner with as many as 5 per cent private patients is unique on the British scene today. An earlier study in 1951–52 estimated that four-fifths of general practitioners had less than twenty private patients.[23]

The number of doctors entirely in private practice is probably at most between 2 and 3 per cent of the total number of active general practitioners.[24] A similar proportion was assumed in 1952.[25] Although statistics on income from private practice are not available, it is obvious that, for most general practitioners in the National Health Service, private practice is not an important source of income.[26] The Minister of Health estimated that for 1962–63 general practitioners in the Service had an average income of £170[27] from non-official sources. This figure included income from other than private practice, but represented less than 8 per cent of average net income.

The proportion of the population who are patients of private practitioners has remained consistently low. In early 1952, 97.7

per cent of a large sample of adults in England and Wales reported that they were registered as National Health Service patients. Included in this group were 2 per cent who also used private practitioners. Of the remainder, 1.5 per cent would use only private practitioners and another 0.2 per cent would probably use private practitioners when ill.[28] In a similar study in 1964, 98.3 per cent of those interviewed were on the list of a National Health Service doctor, and all except 0.8 per cent indicated that they were likely to rely entirely on the National Health Service for medical care. While in both official reports on Health Service lists and studies of practice it cannot be assumed that a completely accurate measure of the population served was obtained, it would be safe to assume that those who use private general practice exclusively would not exceed, and might well be less than, the 3 per cent suggested in the 1964 study.[29]

The data on private practice indicate that, apart from a small proportion of general practitioners and patients, general medical practice is essentially under the National Health Service. The average practitioner has a handful of private patients, and some Health Service patients may occasionally be treated privately by a doctor other than their own. National Health Service doctors receive some income from private or non-official sources, but it is relatively small, and is made up not only of fees from patients treated privately but also from a variety of activities performed for insurance companies and other commercial organizations.

Although the few large surveys conducted since 1948 and the official data of the commissions and the Ministry give a reasonably consistent picture of the relative proportions of National Health Service and private practice, there is little indication of whether private general practice is declining or increasing. Evidence, on the whole, however, points to a declining role for private general practice. Practitioners relying on private practice have on the whole tended to be older than doctors with Health Service practices, and this suggests that many of the former are carrying on practices organized before 1948 while new recruits have gone into the National Health Service.[30] Even among doctors who qualified before 1948, the proportion of those outside the National Health Service has steadily declined since 1949.[31] In 1954, the Fellowship for Freedom in Medicine, which has a large membership of private practitioners, found that a majority of those whom it had polled were of the opinion that private practice had diminished since 1948.[32] Paul Gemmill, as a result of his personal survey, concluded that "private patients are scarce and getting scarcer all the time; so that income from this source is meagre and steadily shrinking."[33] In 1952, the British Medical Association maintained in its negotiations with the Ministry that the original assumption on the part of the Government and itself that 5 per cent of the population would not use the National Health Service, although "the right figure . . . for the first two years of the service," was no longer valid. "The percentage has tended to decrease with the passing of the years."[34]

Hospital and specialist care is the other major component of the Service with a potential for private practice. It is a distinct and separate system, and the nature of private practice within it is affected by factors different from those operating among general practitioners. The possibility of private practice was accepted in the case of general practitioners, but no effort was made to give private practice a formal role in the public scheme. In the case of consultations and specialists, the arrangements for part-time appointments and the provision of private pay-beds in the public hospitals made private practice a recognized part of the National Health Service.

Since a consultant appointment on a hospital staff provides both the prestige necessary for private practice and access to the hospital facilities required for the performance of specialist work, it is likely that the proportion of consultants engaged in part-time hospital work accurately represents private consultant practice. In 1964, of 7,355 paid consultants in the National Health Service hospitals in England and Wales, 5,106 (about 69 per cent) were part-time and 2,249 were whole-time.[35] In 1959, the proportion was 73 per cent, and in 1949, nearly 76 per cent.[36] Although there has been a gradual decline in the proportion of part-time to whole-time consultants in National Health Service hospitals, this in itself is not necessarily indicative of a decline in private consultant practice. Such factors as the appointment of consultants to hospitals in areas where little private practice is available, an increase of the number of consultants in specialties not geared to private practice, and greater prevalence of age groups, i.e., either relatively young or old, for whom private practice is less remunerative than whole-time service, as well as possible administrative pressures toward whole-time service, may suggest that private practice has become a more restricted aspect of consultants' careers.

In its testimony before the Royal Commission on Doctors' and Dentists' Remuneration, the Joint Consultants' Committee, although producing no figures on private consulting earnings, was convinced that there had been a "disastrous" decrease in private practice. The Committee pointed out that the amount of practice varied from area to area and that central London was more fortunate than others in having the patronage of foreign visitors. Specialties, like pediatrics, pathology, and radiology, were particularly marked by the reduction in private practice. The Committee attributed this general decline to the reduction in private hospital beds and their costliness.[37]

The difference in income between part-time and whole-time consultants indicates, however, that the combination of part-time appointment with private practice is still highly remunerative. In 1955–56, the average income of part-time male consultants in Great Britain was £3,603, as compared to £3,002, for whole-timers. It was in the upper part of the income range that the major differences occurred. The highest decile income for part-timers was £5,393 as compared to £3,782 for whole-time consultants. The comparable figure for London part-time consultants was £6,599, or two and one-half times the lowest quartile income for part-timers. Among whole-timers, the differential between the highest decile and lowest quartile income was less than one and one-half times.[38] The higher income range of part-time consultants may be influenced to some extent by the greater prevalence of distinction awards among part-timers. In July 1958, 36.8 per cent of the part-time consultants were receiving such awards as compared to 19.5 per cent of whole-timers. The part-timers were particularly prevalent in the more generous upper categories (A and B awards) where over 15 per cent of the part-timers and less than 5 per cent of the full-timers were represented.[39] Apart from other considerations, the possibility of exceptionally high earnings makes the combination of part-time consultant appointments and private practice a desired goal. This is indicated by the initial preference of part-time to whole-time appointments when, as in many instances, the applicant has the choice, and by the relatively greater transfers from whole-time to part-time status.[40]

As the Joint Consultants' Committee maintained before the Royal Commission, the existence of private consultant practice is critically affected by the availability of private hospital beds. The number of staffed beds allocated to paying patients in the National Health Service in England and Wales has gradually diminished since 1949. In that year the number of Section 5 beds was 6,647; in 1963, the number of such beds allocated was 5,623. During this period the total number of staffed beds in National Health Service hospitals increased from 453,000 to 472,000.[41] In addition to the pay-beds in National Health Service hospitals, there are about 2,900 private-patient beds in voluntary hospitals and nursing homes.[42] At the start of the National Health Service, the government exempted some 250 nursing homes and hospitals from nationalization.[43] The majority of these were run by religious orders and other voluntary bodies, and some were entirely charitable or limited to the use of their membership. Many of the smaller private nursing homes were unable to cope with the demands of modern medical practice and went out of business.[44] Since 1958 the Nuffield Nursing Home Trust, a non-profit body affiliated with the British United Provident Association, the leading voluntary health insurance organization, has acquired, modernized, and built over a dozen private nursing homes with a capacity of 400 beds and plans to expand the number of private beds by almost sixty a year. However, private nursing homes and many of the facilities outside the National Health Service are not of the quality or do not have the resources to satisfy the complex requirements of modern medicine and can only be used selectively by specialists when they are assured of relatively simple and predictable needs on the part of their patients. Thus, the private beds in the National Health Service hospitals are of more than quantitative significance for the private practice of consultants, since they represent the only resource which is fully supported by the necessary staff and equipment.

The proportion of the population using private hospital care is difficult to determine. There is no clear relationship between the private patients of general practitioners and those paying privately for hospital care. Patients may choose to be on a National Health Service doctor's panel and to be treated privately in a hospital or nursing home, or they may choose the reverse. If the experience of the provident societies with insurance for general practice is any indicator, persons providing for hospital costs have little interest in insuring for general practice and may be only limited consumers of private general practice. The provident societies cover around one and one-half million persons, primarily for hospital costs. In 1963, the General Manager of the British United Provident Association estimated that about 50 per cent of admissions to hospital pay-beds and nursing homes were provident subscribers, and assumed, therefore, that some three million or 6 per cent of the population were potential users of private care.[45] This, however, can be considered only a very rough approximation in view of the probably large differences between the insured and non-insured users of private facilities.

CHAPTER 2

Private Health Insurances

PRIVATE health insurance has been ascribed a focal role among those concerned with the maintenance of a private sphere of medicine in Britain. On the practical side, the costs of contemporary medicine could not be borne by consumers without some insurance mechanism; the income and, thus, to a large extent, the existence of private consultant and hospital practice are dependent on the presence of the provident societies.[1] Ideologically, however, the provident societies represent more than the number of subscribers involved. For, although the provident societies have had vast increases in membership since 1948, their total is still relatively small compared to National Health Service patients, and the amount of private expenditure for medicine is a very small proportion of the national health budget. The provident societies, and particularly the British United Provident Association with over 80 per cent of annual subscription income, symbolize the sphere of private practice. Their growth is a measure of the vitality of private medicine and acts as a stimulus to further advance. Like other self-fulfilling phenomena, their growth convinces people of the advantages that must be present in private care and, conversely, of the limitations that must exist within the National Health Service. The very presence of a small but active private insurance movement functions as a locus for dissatisfactions with the public system.

By 1948, when the National Health Service started, hospital insurance was under the aegis of the contributory associations providing free hospital care for low-income groups, while the provident societies met the partial costs of the middle and upper classes. The former, as already noted, had their main start after World War I and vacillated between being charitable collecting agents for the voluntary hospitals and guarantors of hospital care for their low-income subscribers. The provident societies had made a late start and were hardly in operation a decade before the foundations of the National Health Service were laid. Neither the contributory nor provident bodies were in a position to offer a serious alternative to a public scheme.[2]

The contributory and provident societies were faced with a crisis of continued existence. This was particularly true for the former, whose *raison d'être* was the voluntary hospitals which were now to be transferred to public control and support. During the early debates in 1944 on the future health scheme, the then Conservative Minister of Health remarked that the voluntary hospitals could hardly favor the continuance of the contributory schemes merely to maintain the present mode of financing.[3] Many of the contributory societies went out of business, while others lost large sections of their membership. By the end of 1949, it was estimated that the total membership of contributory societies was three million, or less than one-third of the membership before 1948.[4] Some of the leaders of the societies thought of moving in the direction of provident insurance as the Hospital Savings Association had done earlier.[5] While there was some small merging of interests, as in Bristol, in general the two types of societies remained separate. The differences were clearly evidenced at the initial meetings in 1946 of representatives of the provident and contributory societies concerned with the survival of the insurances. That meeting led to the merging of the major provident societies to form the British United Provident Association.[6]

The contributory societies' identification with the working

classes and with the local communities whose hospitals they had served conflicted with the national and upper-class emphasis of the provident societies. At the 1946 meeting, Sir Ernest Rock Carling had explained that the provident societies' role would be related to the needs of private patients in hospitals and nursing homes. He emphasized the need for patients to be cared for in surroundings compatible with their way of life, and hoped that the provident societies would make this possible without anxiety caused by financial difficulties.[7] The functions of the provident and contributory societies were now further apart than they had been before the National Health Service. Previously, both had met hospital costs, although for different income groups. Now that the contributory societies were relieved of the costs of hospital care by free public hospitals, they turned to providing mainly financial sickness benefits to their members. The provident associations, on the other hand, concentrated on insuring members against the costs of private hospital care.

The British United Provident Association was formed in 1947. During its first year it amalgamated with several of the existing provident societies including the Oxford and District Provident Association which brought with it the guarantee of £50,000 for the solvency of the fund which Lord Nuffield had made to that organization. The B.U.P.A. continued its policy of merging with local provident bodies and replacing them with a network of regional offices of its own. By the middle 1960's, the British market was dominated by the B.U.P.A. with the London Association for Hospital Services and the Western Provident Association carrying much smaller lists of subscribers. For the year 1964, the B.U.P.A. had roughly 510,000 subscribers and a subscription income of £6,160,000.[8] The London Association for Hospital Services had 81,000 registered subscribers, and an income of £1,130,000; the Western Provident Association had £265,000 in subscription income and 25,000 members.[9] If dependents covered are included, the total number at risk was about 1,350,000. Even taking into account the changed value of the pound, the growth of the voluntary societies is impressive. In 1949, the combined subscription income of the three societies was less than £190,000 with approximately 50,000 subscribers, and even considering the other provident schemes then existing, the total subscription income could not have been more than £250,000 with 65,000 subscribers. The major growth in the societies occurred after 1954. In their first full five years after the National Health Service started, the three societies reached an annual subscription income of £1,120,000. In 1959, this income had become £4,100,-000 and had grown to an even larger amount by 1964. This great increase in premiums by no means reflected a comparable increase in membership. As will be discussed below, the premium rates have increased considerably over the years. Thus, between 1954 and 1964, the subscription income of the B.U.P.A. increased at more than double the rate of the increase in membership—6.7 compared to 3.1.

The three provident societies, with minor exceptions, provided similar major hospital and consultant benefit plans. Two of the societies, the B.U.P.A. and the Western Provident, have schemes for general practitioner services, but the London Association for Hospital Services, with which the British Medical Association has its group health insurance plan for doctors, has not incorporated such a scheme. The B.U.P.A. introduced its general practitioner plan in January 1959, under pressure from the medical profession, which felt this scheme was essential to the continuance of private practice by general practitioners. Those eligible were limited to subscribers to the B.U.P.A.'s major plan, and the absence of coverage of the cost of drugs was a very significant restriction. The Western Provident scheme also failed to cover drugs. The general practitioner's schemes have made little progress. By June 1965, over four years after the introduction of B.U.P.A.'s scheme, it had only 19,500 registrations or less than 4 per cent of the total subscribers.[10] Pressure continued for the inclusion of drugs in the general practitioner scheme and, at the Annual Representative Meeting of the British Medical Association in July 1964, the Chairman of the Private Practices Committee announced that he was attempting to persuade the B.U.P.A.

to include drugs in their scheme. He stated: "The courage and dedication to the public interest of B.U.P.A. in embarking upon this scheme despite all purely actuarial considerations to the contrary deserve reward and may yet mark a turning point in the affairs of British medicine."[11] Although the B.U.P.A. was giving serious consideration to the matter, up to the summer of 1966 no scheme incorporating payments for drugs prescribed by general practitioners had been established.

The main schemes of the provident societies cover in-patient and out-patient treatment and nursing at home (Table 1). Specifically, the societies pay toward the cost of accommodation in a hospital or nursing home, the fees of physicians, anesthetists, specialists, and surgeons, and the cost of tests and treatment while in a hospital or nursing home. As an out-patient, a subscriber receives payments toward the cost of operations, consultations, tests, and treatment. The insurers contribute toward the fees of a full-time qualified nurse for a patient at home. All of these services must be approved by a doctor. Discretionary grants are generally made if the subscriber receives in-patient treatment as a National Health Service patient. The B.U.P.A. has established maximum limits for each of the separate benefits with no overall maximum. The Hospital Service Plan of the London Association, on the other hand, has (except for its lowest scale) no weekly limit on hospital charges, but sets a maximum for in-patient benefits payable within one year. The B.U.P.A. has a special supplementary scheme restricted to additional benefits for hospital accommodation and nursing. For an additional contribution of between £1 6s. and £3 10s., according to the age of the subscriber and the number of dependents, he may increase his weekly hospital benefit by £6 6s. and his annual hospital benefit by £81 18s. The Western Provident Association has a supplementary cash benefit scheme which offers additional cash benefits unrelated to the cost of treatment.

The cost of hospital accommodation benefits has been a major difficulty for the voluntary insurers. This is the most desired benefit of subscribers who purchase the insurance to obtain the advantage of private hospital care. About 6s. 7d. of benefits are for in-patient costs. In-patient benefits are almost equally divided between hospital or nursing home accommodation charges and professional fees. The B.U.P.A. has had hardly any demand for the *ex gratia* payments which are made to subscribers using hospital facilities as National Health Service patients. Since 1956–57, all special grants including *ex gratia* payments amounted to between 2 and 3 per cent of total claims.[12] The cost of specialist fees for surgery and anesthetics have been controlled by the ceilings for private charges in Health Service hospitals, but the cost of pay-beds has steadily risen. Between 1955 and 1966 (Table 1), the B.U.P.A.'s annual hospital accommodation benefit under the minimal scheme rose from £84 to £382; under the maximum scheme, from £200 to £710. In comparison, total major operation benefits towards surgeon and anesthetist fees rose from £31 to £84 and from £79 to £137, respectively.

The voluntary societies, under these circumstances, have been faced with the problems of marketing insurance with premiums which are sufficiently low to be competitive with a free Health Service, providing benefits adequate enough to be attractive to the public, and at the same time remaining financially solvent. The fact that each of the societies has had at least a dozen schemes on its books since 1948, of which only about one-third are presently in operation, indicates the amount of adjustment required to meet the needs of the market. The London Association, as noted above, reacted to the rising cost of hospital accommodation by removing its ceiling on accommodation charges, but at the same time it compensated for this risk by reducing its yearly maximum in-patient benefits. The B.U.P.A. in 1966 moved from basing its maximum yearly grant for hospital accommodation on a ten-week stay to a thirteen-week stay. This was done without any change in subscription rates although it was accompanied by withdrawal of the lowest scale then in operation and the addition of a higher scale. In view of 1965–66 hospital and nursing home accommodation charges, it was unlikely that any subscriber below Scale 10, the second highest before 1966, would have had

TABLE 1: B.U.P.A. SCALES OF SUBSCRIPTIONS AND BENEFITS

Benefits	1955 Minimum¹ £ s. d.	1955 Maximum² £ s. d.	1960 Minimum¹ £ s. d.	1960 Maximum² £ s. d.	1966 Minimum¹ £ s. d.	1966 Maximum² £ s. d.
Accommodation, Hospital or Nursing						
Home— weekly	8 8 0	19 19 0	17 17 0	42 0 0	29 8 0	54 12 0
yearly	84 0 0	199 10 0	178 10 0	420 0 0	382 0 0	709 16 0
Home Nursing— weekly	4 4 0	8 8 0	6 16 6	18 18 0	12 12 0	22 1 0
yearly	21 0 0	42 0 0	40 19 0	113 8 0	75 12 0	132 6 0
Major Operation, each Fees, Surgeon and Anesthetist	31 10 0	78 15 0	47 5 0	120 15 0	84 0 0	136 10 0
Physician's Fee,— weekly	6 6 0	15 15 0	9 9 0	24 3 0	16 16 0	27 6 0
yearly Hospital or N.H.—	31 10 0	78 15 0	47 5 0	120 15 0	84 0 0	136 10 0
Radiotherapy complete course specialist fee	—	—	44 2 0	105 0 0	75 12 0	115 10 0
Consultation, Pathology, Radiology, Physiotherapy Specialist Fee yearly in-patient full expenses to out-patient	12 12 0³	31 10 0³	18 18 0	46 4 0	31 10 0	53 11 0
half-expenses to yearly	—	—	15 15 0	38 17 0	26 5 0	45 3 0
Subscription Cost— Annual⁴	1 12 6	18 14 0	4 7 0	39 11 0	9 3 0	53 9 0

1. Subscriber, 18–29, without dependents; except 1955: 18–24.
2. Subscriber with two or more dependents, 50 and over; except 1955: 65 and over. In 1960 and 1966, if person 55 or over included at time of joining, subscription raised by 10%; in the 1955 scales there was a special surcharge for inclusion of a person 60 or over.
3. Both in- and out-patients, half expenses paid.   4. Individual subscribers rate.
Note: Schemes have nine subscription categories within each scale, according to age and number of dependents. The two used in Table 1 give range of subscription charges for all scales for the year designated.

his weekly hospital bed cost approximately met.

The B.U.P.A.'s response to the rising cost and alleged shortage of National Health Service pay-beds has been to support the development of nursing homes through the Nuffield Nursing Homes Trust. Early in its history, the B.U.P.A. established Paying Patients' Accommodation Ltd. to stimulate local nursing home accommodation. In 1957, a charitable trust, later to be named the Nuffield Nursing Home Trust, was formed by the Governors of the B.U.P.A. to enter more actively into the provision of private beds. Apart from its organizational support, B.U.P.A. has given solid financial backing to the Nuffield Nursing Homes through interest-free loans, guarantees of loans, and covenants payable out of B.U.P.A.'s investment income. At the launching of the Nursing Home Trust, B.U.P.A. planned to provide deeds of covenant up to £1 million for capital expenditure on nursing home projects. Its current covenant payments are approximately £100,000 annually. By June 1965, it had made interest-free loans of £318,000 to the Trust.[13] The Trust has expected local areas to contribute approximately half of the capital expenditure of homes developed. In addition to maintaining some control over the supply and the cost of private bed accommodation through the Nursing Home Trust, B.U.P.A. also has a financial interest in the use of the nursing homes; this is not the case when its subscribers resort to pay-beds in National Health Service hospitals.

Another serious problem for the provident societies has been the age structure of their subscribers. As might have been expected and as surveys have indicated, private medical care has had a proportionately greater appeal to older people. Younger individuals with lower incomes and family commitments would on financial grounds, if for no other reason, be less amenable to purchasing private health insurance. In the B.U.P.A.'s earliest years, the age limit for joining the scheme was dropped. In 1954, an extra charge of 10 per cent was placed on new subscriptions for those between 60 and 69, and of 20 per cent for those over 70. In 1955, there was a return to the 65 age limit for new subscribers, and during the following years there was a restructuring of the scales towards higher premiums for those in the older age brackets. Currently the B.U.P.A. and the Hospital Service Plan of the London Association have a surcharge for those joining between 55 and 65.

The age distribution of subscribers still remains weighted towards the upper age or high medical risk ages. In the spring of 1965, the ratio of registered B.U.P.A. subscribers aged 50 and over to those 30 to 49 and 18 to 29 was 10:7:3. However, among new registrants in a sample month the ratio was 6:9:5. The encouragement of group schemes has been considered an important influence in changing the age balance of subscribers. In the spring of 1965, the ratio among the three age groups was 4:4:2 among group subscribers and 7:2:1 among individual subscribers. In June 1965, 59.3 per cent of B.U.P.A. subscribers were members of groups. The Hospital Service Plan had approximately 70 per cent of subscribers in business staff and trade and professional groups. In the ten years since 1955, the B.U.P.A. had increased the proportion of its group subscribers from 40 to almost 60 per cent.

One of the major recruitment devices for group schemes has been the rebates allowed members of groups joining the provident societies. The B.U.P.A. allows a 20 per cent rebate for groups where the company is the sponsor but does not contribute toward the cost. Where the company contributes half or more, the reduction is 25 per cent, and in the case of total payment by the company, 33⅓ per cent. The Hospital Service Plan provides somewhat smaller rebates both for company staff schemes and for professional and trade groups. Companies that contribute to the subscriptions of employees can generally charge this as a business expense against profit. British firms have, on the whole, been relatively reluctant to provide fringe benefits of the health insurance type in the past. Studies of firms, conducted around 1960, showed that less than one-third of the larger firms sponsored such insurance, and even among these, expenditures represented less than 0.3 per cent of payroll.[14] Although no exact figures are available, it is likely that company interest in health insurance schemes has expanded, particularly for employees on the professional and management levels and that, in new schemes, companies are making a much larger contribution toward subscription payments. In the autumn of 1965, for example, more than 50 per cent of new B.U.P.A. staff groups, or twice the proportion of old groups, were totally paid for by companies. Reductions, although of a lesser nature, are offered to other groups such as professional and trade organizations. To expedite the formation and administration of group schemes, the B.U.P.A. has established Group Management Ltd. which, for an annual fee of 5s. per member, undertakes all administrative tasks such as publicizing the scheme, collecting subscriptions, and maintaining correspondence related to the group.

The records of the provident societies on the proportion of subscription income returned to subscribers in terms of claims reflects the relative size of the societies. During 1964 and 1965, the B.U.P.A. averaged about 90 per cent of subscription income spent on claims; the Hospital Service Plan, 86 per cent; and the Western Provident Association, 80 per cent. Since 1954–55, the B.U.P.A. has expended between 83 and 92 per cent of current subscription income on claims. In 1964, the Hospital Service Plan sharply cut its administrative costs to 7 per cent, below the B.U.P.A. average of between 9 and 10 per cent in recent years. This has, however, been balanced by higher development costs on the part of the Hospital Service Plan. The B.U.P.A.'s reserves position is impressive. For the year 1964–65, B.U.P.A. had reserves of £2,600,000 or almost 37 per cent of the subscription income and more than 40 per cent of claims for that year. In the past ten years this has increased from £415,000 or just over 25 per cent of subscription income. The large size of these reserves gives the B.U.P.A. a firm position from which to support such ventures as the Nuffield Nursing Homes and the general practitioner scheme. The claims ratio for the latter has always been above 90 per cent and, in 1963–64, it was almost 99 per cent, despite the fact that several first attendances were excluded from payment.

Publicity and marketing are important functions of the provident societies. In 1963–64 and 1964–65, the B.U.P.A. spent £71,000 and £73,000, respectively, or about 1 per cent of subscription income, for development. The Hospital Service Plan spent £59,000 and £37,000 for comparable periods or 6 and 3 per cent, respectively, of subscription income. However, it is difficult to make an accurate comparison of development costs since the B.U.P.A., with its large organization of twenty branch offices, probably has some overlapping between administrative and development costs. In 1965, the Hospital Service Plan had only four branch offices, although it was represented throughout the country by insurance brokers. More and more of the growth of both organizations has been directed to increasing their group membership schemes through contact with firms and other organizations.

The provident societies have, in publicizing their schemes, emphasized the advantages of greater privacy for the patient, the speed and convenience of treatment, and the freedom of choice of the specialist.[15] The concentration on obtaining group memberships, particularly in large firms, has resulted in an emphasis on the value of insurance to the organization.[16] The advantage of this appeal over that to individuals is that it avoids the controversial issue of individual preference or preferred treatment in a democratic welfare society. By placing the onus on the firm's need, private insurance becomes the handmaiden of efficiency and higher productivity and thus enhances social rather than individual goals.

In addition to their own marketing programs the provident societies, and especially the B.U.P.A. and its Nuffield Nursing Homes, have received much publicity from the press. The press coverage was heightened during the autumn of 1965 when interest in the private health and welfare market outside the state services was intensified by the publication of the Institute of Economic Affairs study, *Choice in Welfare*.[17] According to its findings, there was a large public desiring to use private welfare schemes if some form of state subsidy would share in the cost. The idea of choice was not new; it had been debated in the publications of the Bow Group, an unofficial body associated with the Conservative Party. With an election imminent, however, the issue of choice was projected into a major issue of political conflict. Under these circumstances B.U.P.A. and the provident societies were given an important role as viable and growing examples of the principle of choice.

Choice as a relevant issue had been emphasized early after the enactment of the National Health Service by the B.U.P.A. Its early motto was: "If we cherish independence, if we value freedom of choice to pay our own way, it is in times of good health that we make our provision for illness."[18] In the public debate over the issue of choice the provident societies came to stand for more than meeting the desires of a minority of the population seeking to "indulge" themselves in more luxurious medicine. They symbolized for critics of the Health Service its limitations and the desire of an increasing segment of the population for some other form of medicine. The *Financial Times* medical correspondent, on October 2, 1965, after reviewing the benefits of private care and insurance, concluded that "the Minister's antagonism to private practice can only be interpreted as an admission that all is not well with the National Health Service." The B.U.P.A and the other provident societies, which in the past had primarily encouraged those in the medical profession who wished to keep open the door of private care, became important rallying points for critics of the welfare state.

The significance of the growth of the provident societies is difficult to appraise. Their present coverage is still much too small to support the position of those who view their expansion as indicative of a widespread disillusion with the National Health Service. The growing numbers taking out private insurance may not represent any major increase in those using private medical care; indeed it may not involve more than existing consumers of private care going to the insurance market. On the other hand, if private medical insurance becomes an established fringe benefit among companies (a trend the insurance societies are encouraging), this will be an important stimulus to private coverage and may have consequences relevant to both public and private medical care.

While the provident societies have increased their membership and subscriptions since 1948, the contributory associations, whose membership was far greater before the National Health Service, have expanded relatively slowly after their initial setback following the introduction of the public hospital system. In 1964, 37 contributory schemes were functioning with a membership of 4,100,000 and a total subscription income of £3,700,000 as compared to 3,400,000 members and a subscription income of £2,000,000 in 1950.[19] Both of these years must be measured against an estimated 1948 membership of over 10,000,000 with a subscription income of £8,000,000.[20] Since the contributory, like the provident, schemes include dependents, the total numbers currently covered by contributory schemes are probably around 11 million.

With the provision of a free and statutory hospital service, the contributory schemes were faced with the provision of entirely new types of benefits. To a limited extent they maintained their traditional charitable relationship with the hospitals by making small voluntary contributions to local hospitals and encouraging voluntary hospital service by such bodies as the League of Hospital Friends. However, the total contributed to hospitals, since 1948, some £1,300,000,[21] indicates that this is not an important function of the contributory societies. Since the membership of the contributory schemes before 1948 had been limited to low-income groups, they could not appeal to the same desire for private hospital care as had the provident societies. The membership of the contributory societies could not afford the subscription rates required for private treatment nor were they interested in this type of care. The contributory schemes which survived 1948 turned primarily to cash payments during illness as their major benefit. These were expanded by provision of, and reimbursement for, other health needs not supplied or not accessible without cost in the statutory system. Thus, with charge for dentures and glasses in the National Health Service, the contributory societies added some compensation for the expenditures to their schemes. At the end of 1961, the types of benefits provided by contributory societies other than the Hospital Saving Association, in order of their availability, were: convalescent home accommodation, cash benefits during hospitalization, contributions towards glasses, grants for surgical appliances, grants for dentures, payments toward home helps, maternity grants, special consultation grants, physiotherapy, and out-patient grants for those attending spas.[22] The sponsorship of benefits by the societies is influenced by local expectations or traditional policy as well as by the ownership of facilities, like convalescent homes or physiotherapy units, which result in more benefits being channelled toward their maintenance and use.

The proverbial "penny a week" schemes have, on the whole, continued their pre-1948 practice of providing benefits to low-income groups at low cost. For most schemes, the range of contribution is between one and six pennies a week, with three pence as the most common rate. Many schemes have reduced rates for old-age pensioners. The benefits are modest, also. Cash benefits vary extensively among societies. The remaining literally "penny a week" schemes usually have very limited benefits, sometimes only the use of the convalescent home of the society. The average in-hospital maximum cash benefit for the contributor is between twenty and twenty-five pounds a year. Generally, additional grants, although smaller, are made for other members of the family. Some schemes permit higher grants, but limit their occurrence to every second or third year.[23] Some idea of the size of benefits may be obtained from the average payment per claim of the Hospital Saving Association, a wealthy society with an elaborate scheme. For the almost 700,000 claims made between 1963 and 1965, the average payment was £2 12s.[24]

The contributory societies range from smaller locally-based societies with subscription incomes below £20,000 to larger societies such as the Hospital Saturday Fund with an annual subscription income of £275,000 and branch offices throughout the British Isles. The Hospital Savings Associations, the largest, insured about 30 per cent of the over 3 million contributors of the 27 societies affiliated to the British Hospitals Schemes Association in 1962, and its subscription income is well over £1,000,000.[25]

There has been some conflict among the contributory societies between those who view themselves traditionally as inheriting the role of local voluntary charitable societies and those who would expand into the business of sickness insurance. Nearly all still rely on voluntary collecting agents, and the relatively low benefit—contribution ratio compared with the provident societies indicates an acceptance of looser standards of efficiency. However, some of the societies even before 1948 had disregarded local boundaries and moved toward more elaborate insurance schemes. This trend is more noticeable currently when the survival of the smaller schemes appears doubtful and the prosperity of the B.U.P.A suggests that there may be a market for extended benefits among more highly paid workers. Several of the larger societies have introduced the doubling of current schemes as well as more elaborate insurances with expanded benefits.

The subscription rates for these schemes place them well out of the range of conventional contributory societies. The setting of an annual rate in itself symbolizes a sharp break with the traditional weekly collection of pennies. The rates fall between one-third and one-half of the lowest active B.U.P.A. individual scale. Relative to B.U.P.A. benefits, the contributory higher benefit schemes do not appear generous. While the Hospital Saturday Fund offers additional out-patient benefits in the dental and optical areas and a maternity grant, the maximum limits on these benefits keep the cost low. The benefits for hospital and consultant and specialist fees are much less than the provident societies', even taking into account the differences in contribution. Their major advantage over the provident societies is that the contributor receives the hospital benefit whether he is a patient in a public or private bed. Since the hospital benefits, at best, are about one-quarter of weekly charges for private beds and the grants to specialist and consultation fees fall far below the range for serious private treatment, it is not likely that the new contributory schemes, as presently devised, will encourage a significant amount of private treatment. On the other hand, should they become popular, they may provide the foundation for their further extension or create a public who do not identify their health interests entirely with statutory medical services.

Any consideration of the role of non-governmental bodies in insurance should not conclude without some reference to the friendly societies and the trade unions which formed so large a part of the approved societies administering the health insurance program before 1948. Between 1954 and 1964, there was a marked decline in the membership of sickness benefits societies without branches, which account for over two-thirds of friendly society sickness benefits. The total membership dropped by almost 500,000.[26] In 1964, all 9,700 friendly societies, with a membership of 5,700,000, gave a total of £5,500,000 in sickness benefits.[27] In addition, medical aid benefits were provided by some societies. Of the 910 friendly societies without branches, with a membership of 4,500,000, £1,100,000 was spent on medical aid.[28] For friendly societies without branches, sickness benefits, in 1964, were about 20 per cent of total benefits, and medical aid, 6 per cent. In 1954, the proportions were 25 per cent and 5 per cent, respectively.[29] The annual sickness and accident benefits of trade unions were, in 1964, about 5s. per member and twice what they were in 1954, a somewhat greater increase than occurred in other provident benefits provided by trade unions.[30] It is apparent, however, that the former approved societies make a relatively small contribution in sickness and medical aid benefits.

CHAPTER 3

The Patient and Private Practice

W HO are the patients who choose private practice? What segments of the population are consumers of private care? Most studies and observations indicate that private practice appeals primarily to those on the upper income or class range of the socio-economic spectrum. In the early 1950's it was noted in one study that income was the most important factor in distinguishing private patients.[1] Some ten years later, an examination of National Health Service practices showed that in both urban and partly rural areas there was a consistent relationship between income and the amount of private practice, although private practice generally was more common in rural areas. In urban areas, the proportion of doctors with twenty or more private patients varied from 45 per cent in the relatively middle-class sections to 17 per cent in working-class ones. In partly rural areas the proportions were 56 and 29 per cent, respectively.[2]

In rural areas, there has been a greater tendency toward the traditional loyalty to practices established prior to the National Health Service, particularly among the upper classes or the "county families." Thus, there are still "inherited practices" with the continuing patronage of the old aristocracy. However, these groups have been expanded by wealthy business executives who, for social as well as other reasons, emulate the customs of the rural gentry.

A similar weighting of private practice toward the higher income groups appears to occur in hospital care as well. In Cartwright's study of the early 1960's, the middle class put hospital facilities far out of proportion to their numbers in the total sample.[3] The growth of company insurance schemes for management personnel will probably result in a greater usage of private facilities by the upper income urban population. The 1965 survey of the Institute of Economic Affairs indicated that the provident type of insurance was held almost entirely by the upper classes. The lower classes, on the other hand, were generally associated with benefits of the contributory type. Of the 18 per cent of the Institute's sample who had some private insurance, 35 per cent of the upper-middle-class husbands spoke of their insurance as making it possible to obtain a bed and treatment quicker, as compared to 4 per cent of the working class; and 40 per cent of the working class spoke of financial benefits as compared to 8 per cent of the upper-middle and middle classes.[5] It should be noted that although the upper classes tend to make greater use of private hospital, consultant, and general practitioner services, there is no evidence that on the whole they are making less use of the public services. In fact, all indications appear to the contrary.[6]

Age, possibly associated with income and class, has been found to be most closely connected with private care, particularly in general practice. Many of the people on the private list of practitioners are older patients who were formerly the private patients of these practitioners before the National Health Service or who have been with the same doctor over very lengthy periods.[7] The children of these patients frequently, however, join the National Health Service when they become financially independent of their parents.[8] Older patients, whose habits with respect to medical practice were established before 1948, may prefer a paying relationship with the doctor, and some older patients with greater need for medical attention may feel more comfortable as private patients because of their greater demands on the doctor's time.

Conventional views of medical practice generally have influenced preference for private medicine. Reasons of ideology or custom may keep people from joining a National Health Service list. Those who strongly oppose the National Health Service and the welfare state may tend more than others to resort to private medical care, but they may feel even more eligible for public benefits in response to their heightened consciousness of the tax burden. Traditional attitudes toward medical practice, loyalty to particular medical practitioners and consultants, and unfamiliarity or discomfort with the terms of the National Health Service, by no means account for all who choose to pay rather than use the free public service. There are other advantages which many seek to obtain from the private purchase of medical care, although it should be noted that the largest proportion of those making some private insurance provision in 1965 were in the older age group and referred to their pre-Health Service attitudes as a major reason for the present private provision.[9]

Arranging for medical attention according to one's own time or convenience is frequently stressed by those under private medical care. In private general practice, appointments are made to suit the schedule of the patient rather than the organization of the doctor's practice. In some practices, only private patients are met by appointment; the remainder are treated in the order of waiting during general office hours in the morning and evening. Not only is attention given at a time convenient to the patient, but the physician may make a home visit in circumstances where he would expect the public patient to come to the office. The physician may also give the private patient some tests and treatment for which he would ordinarily refer his National Health Service patient to the hospital.

Although the convenience of timing may be important to the patient of the general practitioner, it is chiefly stressed in relation to hospital treatment. Other than for urgent cases, there may be a long delay in admission to hospitals for surgery and treatment, and the patient is dependent on the hospital's own schedule for the timing of his admission. The private patient, however, relies on the private beds in National Health Service hospitals or in nursing homes which are directly controlled by the private consultant whose patient he is. This is considered particularly advantageous for executives and important business personnel whose stay in hospital can be arranged in accordance with their organization's needs. As mentioned earlier, this is one of the major inducements used to persuade companies to pay for the private insurance of their employees. The consultant's influence over the scheduling of National Health Service free beds sometimes has the result that patients who do not wish to enter a hospital as paying in-patients arrange for private out-patient consultations in the hope that this will expedite hospital admission. Such conduct is strongly denounced by the Ministry of Health, and the profession officially denies that private consultations may be used for "jumping the queue" for National Health Service beds. Patients and general practitioners, however, recognize that the patient who has had a consultation (and a private consultation can be arranged with less delay) may have the informal advantage of interesting the specialist sufficiently to speed his hospital admission.[10] The private out-patient consultation may, also, secure for the patient the consultant's attention after he is admitted. This is particularly important to the patient in surgery since National Health Service patients are usually dependent on the hospital staff for selection of their surgeon. The choice of consultant or specialist, is, of course, one of the major privileges for which the private hospital patient is willing to pay.

Patients, like doctors, are often not fully private. Some services may be used privately, or on particular occasions the patient may make use of private attention although the greater part of his care is under the National Health Service. In general, however, the division between public and private, when it occurs, is a health service general practitioner and private hospital care. Sometimes families will be divided, with most members on a Health Service panel and one or two using a private practitioner. In other situations, persons on a panel may use another doctor privately or may turn occasionally to a private practitioner for a second opinion.

Although the use of two doctors is often complicated, it can be exacerbated under the conditions of the National Health Service. Patients may feel uneasy at officially withdrawing from the panel of a doctor and may continue with him despite their lack of confidence. They then may rely more or less regularly on private attention. This can create difficulties for doctor-patient relationships and relationships between doctors.

More serious from a legal as well as an ethical point of view is the possible collusion between a National Health Service and a private practitioner in the supply of drugs to a private patient. Since the major financial barrier to seeking private attention in general practice is the cost of drugs, arrangements have sometimes been made for the private patient of one doctor to obtain his prescriptions as the National Health Service patient of another. It is also possible, where some members of a family are National Health Service patients and others are private patients of the same doctor, for prescriptions for the latter to be made in the name of the former.[11]

The use of private medical care, whatever its rationale in concrete benefits, cannot be entirely divorced from satisfactions of status or prestige. The patient frequently may get no different medical care than he would under the National Health Service, or very little to reflect the difference in cost. In some cases, as in the use of private nursing homes, the patient may be taking a greater medical risk than if his treatment were undertaken in a National Health Service hospital. It is difficult to separate much of the motivation for private medical care from a desire for what is believed to be the additional social status of private attention.[12]

The question of two class systems of medicine arose early in the debates on the National Health Service. Its opponents made a vigorous attack on the possibilities for private practice included in the bill. Bevan, although agreeing in principle stated that it was "impossible to legislate for snobbishness," and since doctors might believe it worthwhile to remain entirely outside the Service to obtain the advantages of private practice, it might be better to tolerate private practice within the Service and let "middle class people . . . pay them fees."[13]

The position of being a private patient, in itself, distinguishes the patient, at least in his own eyes, from the mass of National Health Service patients. There is no evidence that this feeling is shared by any large number of National Health Service patients. A recent study of patients showed that only six per cent of such patients might seek private general practice if they could afford it.[14] The treatment of the private patient by those in the medical profession who seek to encourage private practice and the publicity of the provident societies both subtly and directly cater to status satisfactions. This is probably most apparent in general practice where the concrete advantages of avoiding the waiting list for a Health Service bed or a private room are not available. In general practice, the physician gives the private patient a more dominant or controlling role than he permits in his National Health Service practice. He is often willing to see the patient when the patient wants, where the patient wants, and as frequently as the patient wants. The physician is generally willing to give the patient much more of his professional time even when he is not convinced of its medical necessity. This contrasts particularly with National Health Service practice where many doctors have concentrated on the most efficient administration of their own professional time and energy in terms of the needs of a large practice list. In effect, the private patient in return for his fee may expect and receive some reversal of prevalent practice. As one general practitioner stated:

Patients must realise that, with the National Health Service they cannot have it all their own way. If the service is to work, they have got to co-operate with the doctor. If they want unnecessary visits, then I tell them straight out they have to become private patients.

The consultant, too, gives the private patient more of his own personal attention and time, but he has the advantage that the patient gains prestige by merely being the patient of the 'great man'. The privacy of the consulting-rooms in Harley Street or wherever the consultant has his office is of importance to the patient. If he is in a hospital, a private bed gives the patient status and privileges. A nursing home may have an even greater aura of respectability as it has a select clientele and avoids the charitable and poor law connotations which have been historically associated with the term hospital on the British scene.

CHAPTER 4

Issues for Private Practice

DURING the decades since the establishment of the National Health Service there has arisen a large variety of issues affecting directly or indirectly the position of private practice. The declarations and actions of professional societies, such as the British Medical Association and more particularly the small but articulate Fellowship for Freedom in Medicine, and the testimony before commissions and committees have, at times, magnified the significance of the issues related to private practice. Although the question of private practice is still of concern in policy-making for the Health Service, it is not of focal or central importance among those officially responsible for the service and among those who represent the interests of the medical profession. The issues affecting private practice under the National Health Service may be divided into three broad categories: (1) services for patients; (2) the balance between private and National Health Service functions in medical practice; and (3) broad proposals for reorienting the relationship between public and private responsibility for the health services.

Services for Patients

Perhaps the most salient issue between the government and those interested in the maintenance of private practice has been the supply of drugs to private patients on the same terms as National Health Service patients. As noted above, the medical profession under the leadership of the B.M.A. interpreted the government's policy in 1946 as permitting the use of any or all of the services, thus making possible the combination of private general medical care and National Health Service prescribing. Bevan, on the other hand, as the first Minister of Health for the National Health Service took the position that, under Section 38 of the Act, "prescription and provision must be treated as part of one process" and that these could not be separated to allow a general practitioner who had no responsibility for the patient under the National Health Service to make drugs available as if he had.[1] Bevan's interpretation of Section 38 has not been questioned by future governments, whether Labour or Conservative, and it has been assumed that any change of policy would require an amendment of Section 38 of the National Health Service Act. In 1950, in response to pressures from those who supported and those who opposed the unity of general medical service and drugs, Bevan indicated that it would be clearly illegal for a doctor to treat privately and prescribe publicly.[2] In 1956, the General Medical Council severely admonished a doctor who had been supplying private patients with National Health Service drugs on the grounds that they could not afford to pay for their drugs, and recommended that the doctor be heavily fined.[3] However, as already noted, a variety of subterfuges may be used for obtaining drugs for private patients, and it was estimated in 1956 that over 50 per cent of private patients were registered with National Health Service doctors for the sole purpose of obtaining prescriptions.[4]

From 1948 onward, the British Medical Association has continuously pressed for National Health Service drugs to be made available to private patients. Regularly, the Annual Representative Meeting of the B.M.A. has reasserted this policy and charged the leadership to take steps to bring about its implementation. By the 1960's, there was a noticeable impatience among some delegates to the Annual Meeting with the lack of progress. A motion was presented in July 1961, although later withdrawn, which voiced "grave concern [at] the Council's lack of success in obtaining National Health Service drugs for private patients." It was suggested that "the collaboration policy of the Council as advocated by the Chairman of the Private Practices Committee" was "mainly to blame" and "a more forceful policy" was demanded.[5] Again, at the time of the very sensitive negotiations between the B.M.A. and the government in 1965, the absence of any reference to drugs for private patients in the "Charter" the policy statement of the B.M.A., was noted in the Council. It was finally agreed that rather than including drugs among the imperative issues of the negotiations, a separate communication would be sent to the Minister of Health making the Association's position clear.[6]

The reluctance of the leadership to view drugs for private patients as of primary concern to the interests of the total medical profession was openly supported by at least some of the membership. Although the correspondence columns of the British Medical Journal and its Supplement were generally filled by supporters of National Health Service drugs for private practice, there were those who questioned this policy.[7] In 1959, the opinion was expressed by one doctor that "an enormous amount of time and effort seems to have gone into the question of free drugs for private patients, [and] is it not like flogging a dead horse?" He continued:

Anyone can sense that private practice has "had it," so why try to resurrect it? Even the rich flock to the surgery, for their rep. mist. The poorer folk often lament they "would rather pay," but look back to the days of private practice, and how often did they pay? The rich were soaked to offset this, but nowadays the apparently rich are not so blooming rich.[9]

At the Annual Representative Meeting in July 1964, it was suggested that the traditional policy on drugs was no longer realistic, that its discussion at meetings merely used up valuable time, and that, at best, some compromise proposal might be made whereby private patients would pay some proportionate charge for drugs. Even the Fellowship for Freedom in Medicine, staunchly identified with the cause of private practice, had suggested the possibility of an alternative to giving private patients exactly the same rights as National Health Service patients.[9] However, the Representatives refused to accept defeat and decided to continue with the traditional drug policy.[10] Some even supported the taking of unilateral action in supplying patients with drugs.[11]

One of the great disappointments of the advocates of drugs for private patients was the failure of the Conservatives during their lengthy period of power to reverse Bevan's policy. The Conservatives, in 1949, had pledged themselves to a new drug policy, but when they came into power several years later they did not feel called upon to fulfill their earlier promise.[12] During its period of office, the Conservative government never directly opposed the principle of drugs for private patients, and at times it lent a sympathetic ear to those in favor, but all the same, it gave no more active support than the previous Labour government. At the end of 1960, over 170 Conservative back-benchers laid down a motion in the House urging the government to introduce legislation for the provision of drugs to private patients.[13] The Minister had already given consideration to the matter, and in November 1959 stated the government's policy:

The Government attach importance to the preservation of private practice and the right of patients to resort thereto, and would certainly consider making drugs available to private patients on National Health Service terms, in the context of available resources and competing claims, if it were shown that the present position was endangering the existence of private practice or preventing any substantial number of people from availing themselves of it, who would otherwise do so. But they have no present plans for legislation on this subject.[14]

The return of a Labour government only brought further discouragement. The Chairman of the Private Practices Committee of the B.M.A. wondered whether it was even worth pursuing the matter with the government. However, as already noted, the issue was brought to the attention of the Minister of Health during negotiations for a new contract between the government and the doctors. In his response, the Minister clearly showed his opposition to any proposal not only for drugs, but for the encouragement of private practice. He favored the doctors' persuading people "to make use of the social services which the community has provided." He felt that the private patient already has the advantage of "a special claim on his doctor's time." He concluded:

> My object—and I am sure the B.M.A. shares it—is to raise the standard of general practice under the service to such a level that ultimately there will be no benefit to patients seeking private treatment. I feel certain even then, private general practice will continue in being, and it is certainly no part at all of my intention to stop it, but if it were at a rather lower level than now I should not regard this as a hardship to either patients or doctors.[15]

Despite philosophical differences about the place of private practice, the grounds used by both Labour and Conservative governments in opposing the provision of drugs to private patients were fundamentally similar. Both were concerned with the problem of controls over prescribing when the patient and physician were outside the National Health Service, the related difficulty of increasing costs arising from prescribing for private patients, and finally the possibility of encouraging the development of two standards of medicine, public and private. At the start, the government relied primarily on the issue of controls. Bevan stated, in 1948, that a doctor serving private patients "would have no responsibility for observing the general conditions which govern prescribing at public expense,"[16] and gave the same reason some two years later when questioned in Parliament.[17] In 1954, the report of the Central Health Services Council's Committee on General Practice in the National Health Service—the Cohen Committee—rejected the idea of National Health Service prescriptions for private patients because it had come to the conclusion that the doctors would not submit to government controls.[18]

The Minister of Health accepted the Committee's recommenda-
tion on the administrative difficulties in ensuring adequate
supervision of private prescribing.[19]

The medical profession immediately reacted by denying that
the problem of controls was insurmountable. In 1956, the B.M.A.
surveyed 573 general practitioners "thought to be engaged solely
in private practice." Of these, 448 would and 30 would not use a
scheme for the provision of drugs to private patients; 434 would
agree and 44 would not agree "to submit to reasonable safeguards
negotiated between the Ministry and the B.M.A.;" and 408 would
and 70 would not "agree to be liable to any penalty imposed
under the terms of safeguards."[20] By 1959, the B.M.A. was willing
to accept most of the terms suggested by the Ministry, and there
was general agreement about the registration of private patients
and doctors and the possible sanctions to be imposed should any
doctors not fulfill their obligations.[21] The government, however,
did not see its way to implementing the scheme although the
B.M.A. had broadly accepted its terms.

This unwillingness was due to two major obstacles—the cost
and the political implications of responsibility for fostering private medicine. The question of administrative controls had been
a convenient excuse, but when it was no longer present, the other
or underlying issues came to the fore. The British Medical Association and the Fellowship for Freedom in Medicine pointed to
the potential savings to the government of providing drugs for
private patients. Many private patients were currently getting
their drugs as Health Service patients. In the long run, there
would be a great saving if private patients could obtain drugs on
National Health Service terms as private practice was more effective and more economical in the use of drugs.[22] Patients and doctors in private medicine, it was also maintained, saved the state
capitation fees and pension allowances, respectively.

The Treasury, however, failed to be convinced by these argu-
ments. Throughout the period, the Minister of Health, whether
Conservative or Labour, eventually referred to the annual cost
(estimated in 1959 as £2¼ million and in 1965 as £3 million with

a "strong probability" of rising) and the fact that the government could not give "high priority" to the drug scheme.[23] Apart from the financial costs, the political costs were potentially high. Although private practice might appeal to some in principle, the vast majority of patients and doctors had little to gain from it and might be antagonized by a scheme which might seem to benefit a small minority at the cost of the majority. As one doctor remarked, "Why should the taxpayer subsidize the private patients?"[24] The issue was put bluntly by Sir Henry Cohen in explaining the opposition to drugs for private patients of the Central Health Service Council's Committee on General Practice:

If you allow patients who pay their doctor a fee privately to have drugs under the National Health Service you are creating within the National Health Service two standards of general practice, with all the disadvantages thereof. . . .[25]

The B.M.A. and the Fellowship for Freedom in Medicine pointed to the advantages of competition within the medical service,[25] but they were not sufficiently convincing to persuade either party to support their cause.

To what extent the expense of drugs acts as a deterrent to those interested in becoming private patients is difficult to determine. Drugs account for over one-third of the cost of general medical care to private patients.[27] There might be some increase in the number of private patients if drugs were provided, but it is unlikely that there would be "a vast exodus of patients away from treatment under the National Health Service."[28] While much has been made of the effects of the drug policy,[29] there is no indication of a significant untapped reservoir of people anxious to become private patients. Surveys have shown relatively small proportions of the population dissatisfied with present care under the National Health Service,[30] and there is no evidence that even the dissatisfied would turn to private practice. It is interesting to note that in July 1951 a small sample of doctors were equally divided in their opinions about whether drugs were a factor in influencing people to avoid private practice.[31] On the other hand, the provision of drugs for private patients might encourage doctors to persuade patients, whom they otherwise would not accept, to come to them as private patients.

While the issue of drugs for private patients absorbed the attention of those concerned with maintaining private general practice, the questions of pay-beds for private hospital patients was of even greater import to the large numbers of consultants and specialists who received a substantial income from private practice. In introducing the National Health Service Bill, in 1946, the government had merely given general approval to family doctors "to make private arrangements for treating such people as still wish to be treated outside the service."[32] However, the treatment of private hospital patients was made an integral part of the Service. "Separate pay-bedrooms or blocks" were to be provided "for which people can pay the whole cost privately and in which part-time specialists within the service can treat private patients."[33] Bevan, answering critics of the establishment of private beds in the public hospitals, maintained that if such beds were not provided there would be a growth of private nursing homes and specialist practice outside the National Health Service, and he supported the "principle" of "relating prices to differences in accommodation.[34]

Under Section 5 of the Act, the Minister was authorized to set aside hospital accommodation for patients who would pay for the full cost of their treatment. Two types of patients were indicated, those under Subsection (1) who would have no private contract with a consultant or specialist and would pay total costs to the hospital, and those under Subsection (2) who had contracted privately for their specialist services and would pay for this service separately in fees to the consultant or specialist. The Joint Committee of Consultants and Specialists representing the profession were of the opinion that medical practitioner service would not be provided unless the patient had an arrangement of his own under Subsection (2),[35] and, in fact, Subsection (1) had been inoperative, for all practical purposes.[36] Thus, all patients in private beds have been the private patients of specific specialists.

The specialists who use the private beds for their patients are generally those with part-time appointments on the hospital staff. In principle, anyone on the medical staff of a hospital in the Service may make use of the private beds in any health service hospital. In practice, the beds are controlled by the senior staff within the hospital and there is little likelihood of any other doctor's using such beds for his private patients.[37]

The problem of allocation of beds was a difficult one. The Ministry desired to provide enough beds for private patients and for National Health Service patients wanting more privacy "without detriment to the facilities required by non-paying patients needing urgent admission, privacy, or isolation on medical grounds.[38] At the start of the Service before it could make a proper survey of hospital accommodation generally, the Ministry continued the number of private beds existing before the Act—some 2 per cent of the total.[39] By March 1949, schemes submitted to the Minister by the Regional Hospital Boards indicated that there would be some reduction in the total number of private beds.[40] Since 1949, there has been a gradual reduction of staffed beds allocated for private patients, from 6,647 to 5,623 in 1963. The major reduction in private beds occurred before 1955. Both the numbers and the proportion of total staffed beds since that time have remained relatively constant, approximately 1.2 per cent.[41]

The medical profession, and particularly the part-time consultants, have been critical of what they considered to be an inadequate number of private beds and the high charges imposed on private patients for the use of these beds. Both these factors, they maintain, have discouraged the growth of private hospital practice. The British Medical Association and its Central Consultants and Private Practice Committees have continually pressed the Government to increase the number of beds and to reduce the charges, and the representatives of the Royal Colleges have been involved through the Joint Consultants' Committee. In 1962 and 1963, there were six meetings of this Committee with the Ministry on the problem of private beds.[42] The concern about the number of beds in the Health Service hospitals was exacerbated by the diminishing number of private beds outside the service. Nursing homes did not have the financial resources to continue, and although the Nuffield Nursing Home Trust had endeavored to increase the amount of private accommodation, it was believed that there were insufficient private funds to meet the need.[43]

The complaints of shortages in private beds in National Health Service hospitals were not confirmed to the Ministry's reports on occupancy rates. The daily occupancy rate by paying patients of pay-beds between 1953 and 1963 had been about 50 per cent.[44] Before 1953, the rate had been lower.[45] The occupancy rate of the beds themselves had been higher because they had been used, at times, for non-paying patients. With the latter, the rate rose to approximately 70 per cent for the period.[46] This may be compared to a better than 85 per cent average occupancy rate for all National Health Service beds during the period 1953–1963.[47]

The B.M.A., however, maintained that the average occupancy rate of pay-beds for the country as a whole was not a valid indicator of the situation. Although the number of beds in some areas was adequate and in some even greater than the demand, there were others in which it was "grossly inadequate."[48] An analysis by Lees and Cooper emphasized the variable nature of the supply of beds. In 1960, they pointed to the variation between 43.4 occupancy rate in all regional boards and the rate of 73.6 per cent for paying patients in London teaching hospitals. They considered the low occupancy rate to be influenced by the small number of beds in some hospitals and their unavailability when there were shortages of staff.[49] The Central Consultants' Committee also criticized the conditions of the beds and said that, in some instances, they were so poor that doctors would not allow their patients to use them. The opinion was expressed that facilities for private patients should be on the level of a "first-class, four-star hotel."[50]

Throughout the period, however, successive Ministers of Health were concerned about the low occupancy rate of private beds. After examining the figures for 1952 and 1953, a Conservative Minister instructed the hospitals to fill vacancies with non-paying patients.[51] In 1966, the Minister of Health asked all hospital boards to review the pay-bed situation in their hospitals. He mentioned the low occupancy rate as compared to other beds, and while he recognized that there would be some difference, he felt that the large existing differences had resulted in "paying patients being able to gain admission more speedily than non-paying patients with similar medical needs." When the occupancy rate by paying patients was below 50 per cent, the Minister would expect some reduction, and even when it was higher a reduction might be necessary in view of the pressure on ordinary National Health Service beds.[52]

The cost to private patients of hospital care was also the subject of much disagreement between the government and those interested in private hospital care. The cost of pay-beds had risen continuously since 1948, and there was strong feeling that this had discouraged many who might be private patients. The cost varied according to the individual cost figures of the hospitals in which the beds were located. Thus, there were differences, for example, between small provincial hospitals and the London teaching hospitals. In 1958, hospital bed costs to private patients varied from between £14 and £19 per week in small country hospitals to between £26 and £38 in London teaching hospitals.[53] In 1965, the range was from £30 to £35 per week in provincial teaching and non-teaching hospitals and up to £45 in London teaching hospitals.[54] The critics of hospital bed costs complained about the accounting techniques used in the hospitals, but they were primarily disturbed by the inclusion of charges which they thought were inappropriate because some of the items were for services not relevant to private patients.

The cost of pay-beds was reduced in 1953 by excluding charges for some services considered not to be of benefit to private patients, and both the surcharges over ward costs as well as the base on which they were calculated were lowered.[55] In 1958, however, a new method of calculating charges resulted in a sizable increase in the cost of pay-beds. There was continued criticism of the items used in calculating the cost of pay-beds, and the sur-charge was attacked as being "out of all proportion to the addi-tional cost of running a private bed as compared with a public bed."[56] In 1966, the Minister informed the House of Commons that he planned to change the basis of accounting hospital charges from individual hospital costs to different classes of hospitals on a national scale.[57]

Although the B.M.A., the Fellowship for Freedom in Medicine, and the consultants were of the opinion that the estimates of pay-bed costs were too high, there were those who felt the real cost was higher than that fixed by the hospitals. The conflict was not so much with the originally calculated cost figures as with the greatly rising cost of current hospital facilities. In 1950, Bevan noted that the cost of private beds almost doubled, but pointed to increased hospital costs generally as the reason. Despite the rise in the cost of pay-beds, the income to the hospitals from private in-patients remained almost a constant proportion of total National Health Service hospital expenditures between 1951–52 and 1961–62, (0.8 to 0.9 per cent).[58] The cost of accommodation in private nursing homes was close to Health Service charges; only in homes run by religious orders were the costs considerably lower.[59]

Advocates of private hospital care have suggested that the prin-ciple of "full" cost be abandoned and that hospital costs be cal-culated so that pay-beds are not so expensive as to be out of the reach of all but a small minority. The Porritt Committee in its report to the B.M.A., the Joint Consultants' Committee in their testimony before the Royal Commission on Doctors' and Dentists' Remuneration, and witnesses before the Guillebaud Committee, all proposed that some figure below cost should be set for pay-beds.[60] In general, the argument for reduced cost rested on the assumption that the private patient would otherwise have occu-pied a free Health Service bed and that this saving to the service should be taken into account when establishing the charge for pay-beds.[61] The growing membership of the provident societies has been pointed to as evidence of a large middle-class demand for private beds, and the consultants suggested to the Ministry in 1963 that moderately priced private beds be provided for people of modest means.[62]

The proponents of reduced charges have received little support in official channels. Other than the 1953 readjustment of charges, there has been no effort to keep down the cost of pay-beds. In 1963, the Minister of Health under a Conservative Government rejected the suggestion of the Joint Consultants' Committee for reduced charges to private patients because, as he stated, it was not "possible to justify subsidising from the Exchequer patients who have chosen to have private treatment."[63] The Guillebaud Committee maintained that a reduction in charges would have to be very substantial before a significant increase in demand would occur, and this would entail a loss to the Treasury.[64] To deal with the problem of low occupancy of pay-beds and the demand for private accommodation, however, it recommended what has been generally accepted policy, the use of pay-beds for non-paying patients and the encouragement of greater use of amenity beds for those willing to pay a small charge for additional privacy.[65]

While the rising charges for pay-bed accommodation were worrying those interested in private hospital care, the statutory schedule of fees which limited the amount specialists and consultants could charge private hospital patients was also a source of irritation. Although the government had opened the door to private specialist practice in the hospitals in the 1946 Act, it had established controls on specialist charges "to prevent the sheer abuse of hospital facilities placed at his [the specialist's] disposal."[66] When the Act went into effect in July 1948, the government had a detailed fee schedule which set maximum fees for classified types of treatment and care. Surgical operations were divided into three classes, major, intermediate, and minor, and the types of operations falling under each of these classes were exhaustively listed. Maximum fees were given for each of the classes and an overall limit of 75 guineas was set for the charges which could make for "one series of treatments of a patient for relief of the same condition." If more than one physician was involved, the fees would be divided within the 75 guinea maximum.[68] Fifteen per cent of accommodation was exempted from these limits.[69]

Criticism soon arose among specialists and consultants that the schedule had not kept up with increasing costs. The specialists desired either total abandonment of the fee schedule or a looser system which would permit charges related to the patient's financial circumstances.[70] In 1953, the Minister, although sympathetic to the specialists' demands, felt he could not abolish the schedule. "Whatever might happen in the future," he said, "the time is not ripe for that."[71] The Minister made some small modifications in the schedule. The overall charges for one treatment were raised to 125 guineas under certain circumstances, and maximum charge for several consultations and attendances, not involved in surgery, were increased from 25 to 40 guineas.[72]

The consultants continued to express their dissatisfaction with the fee schedule, and in many instances, the fee schedules were not followed. In two years, for example, the Western Provident Association reported recovering some £1,700 for 110 of their subscribers because of overcharges.[73] In view of the relatively small size of the Western Provident Association, if similar overcharges were generally prevalent the total would indicate a significant evasion of the schedule. Although the major provident societies, the B.U.P.A. and the Hospital Service Plan, have recognized that there have been abuses of the fee schedule they have preferred to take no action or have resorted to informal pressures.[74] As the Chairman of the B.U.P.A. suggested to the medical profession, "If private practice is to survive, fees and charges must be kept to the minimum. The position of the private patient is too precarious for fancy fees."[75]

On the whole, the Ministry of Health has not been too vigorous in surveillance of specialist charges. Hospital regulations require that a private patient be informed of alternative forms of care available and of the potential charges under the fee schedule. It is hospital policy to have the patient sign a contract which either requires adherence to the schedule or waives the schedule and permits the physician to fix his own charges.[76] The Ministry's emphasis on the patient's being given a clear understanding of the care for which he is eligible under the Health Service and the expenses entailed in private care resulted from "many members of the public" having "a feeling that they have been unfairly treated and have incurred charges either unnecessarily or in excess of what they expected."[77] The hospital may arrange to collect the private professional fee of the specialist at the same time as the hospital charge. This is at the discretion of the specialist who must pay a small deduction to cover administrative expenses. The hospital, however, accepts no responsibility to see that the specialists' fees are paid under any circumstances.[78] In the experience of the Western Provident Association, specialists who collected their fees through the hospitals made charges within the fee schedule, but the schedule tended to be overlooked by physicians and surgeons who charged their patients directly. The Ministry's position has been that if a patient has been overcharged, it is a matter between the patient and his specialist.[79]

On the whole, the Ministry has shown little enthusiasm for enforcing the fee schedule. Although some officials have felt that the Health Service hospitals should not be used for excessive professional profits and fees should be controlled, the fee schedule has operated more as an abstract than as an effective standard. The fact that the Ministry did not revise the schedule after 1953 indicated that it did not look to it as a realistic control. The Ministry shared the viewpoint of the medical profession which was of the opinion that "the fee to be charged should be a private matter for arrangement between the patient, the general practitioner, and the consultants."[80] The B.U.P.A., probably the major single contributor to private professional fees, favored abolition of the fee schedules because of their ineffectiveness.[81] Other provident executives also pointed to the large proportion of patients using private hospitals and nursing homes where the rates were already a good deal higher than the Ministry's ceilings.[82] The larger provident societies had independently established their own schedules for meeting the cost of medical services to their subscribers. The Minister of Health in January 1966, outlining his plans for the immediate future, mentioned among other proposals related to private hospital care, his intention to abandon fee limits.[83]

The issue of private hospital care has been much more hotly contested than the continuation of private general practitioner practice. Private hospital care is much more visible than the services of the family doctor. Although there may be a scarcity of the latter and that which exists is over-used, the waiting lists for hospital beds and the evident quicker attention given private patients have kept private beds a salient issue. As compared to private general practice, the state had made available to private specialist practice an extremely expensive and valuable public commodity: hospital accommodation and resources. There has been much criticism of the way these hospital facilities have been used in private practice. Bevan, in 1953, said that he had introduced pay-beds to keep the specialists in the hospitals, but now they had developed a vested interest in private beds and had abused the provision of Section 5 by restricting their use and keeping them empty so that they might be immediately available when desired by the specialist.[84]

From the start of the Service, private hospital beds had not been popular with many Labour members of Parliament. Bevan's analogy of a theatre with different priced seats was not considered appropriate. Although Bevan's strategy of winning over the consultants and specialists was appreciated, there was strong opposition to the idea of two classes of hospital patients. The Labour Party Executive, in 1954, resolved to abolish pay-beds. In the words of their spokesman, "We believe that jumping the queue in anything is wrong, but jumping the queue where sickness is concerned really goes against all the best instincts of decent people."[85] Although the Labour Party continued to oppose the presence of private accommodation in National Health Service hospitals, the demand for their immediate abolition became less urgent. As with other aspects of the service, it was hoped that improvements in the state scheme would obviate the need for anyone to resort to private care.[86] The Minister's 1966 proposals, however, indicated a more restrictive policy toward private practice in hospitals. In addition to a possible reduction in the number of pay-beds as a result of the projected occupancy survey, the Minister has also suggested that where pay-beds are distributed in small number over several hospitals it might be well to concentrate them while at the same time reducing their numbers.[87] This may have the effect of withdrawing private practice from some areas, discouraging part-time specialists from seeking appointments with several hospitals for the use of their beds, and greater administrative controls and more efficient use of private care.

In principle, Conservative governments were inclined to be favorable to private medical provision and private hospital practice.[88] There was, however, little that the Conservative governments did to expand the field of private hospital practice. The Central Consultants and Specialists Committee and the Private Practices Committee of the B.M.A. were so frustrated in their negotiations with the Ministry that they doubted whether the government really wanted to continue private practice.[89] The position of the Guillebaud Committee, in 1956, probably summarizes the major area of agreement of both parties on the question of private beds.

Whilst appreciating the reasons why some have objected to the provision of pay-beds, we do not ourselves believe that the objections are strong enough to warrant the abolition of pay-beds in the hospital service. If there is any 'jumping of the queue' it cannot amount to very much when account is taken of the relatively small number of pay-beds at present provided in hospitals. In our view a more important issue is that hospital authorities should not keep beds empty any longer than is absolutely necessary. . . .
We accept, therefore, the provision of private accommodation in National Health Service hospitals, both for patients who need it on medical grounds and those who are prepared to pay for it, either in the form of an amenity bed or a pay bed. So long as the present shortage of hospital accommodation continues, however, we would deprecate any expansion in the number of amenity beds and

pay beds which would be at the expense of the available free beds in the service.[90]

The Balance Between Private and National Health Service Practice

The National Health Service, although established to provide full medical services of high quality for the total population, recognized the possibility of some doctors dividing their services between the National Health Service and private practice. For consultants, the organization of a range of part-time scales institutionalized a system of divided practice. For the general practitioner, the situation was more complicated. Since there was no fixed standard of full-time employment, the balance of time allotted to public and private practice was largely up to the discretion of the individual doctor. Unlike the consultant, the general practitioner could remain totally outside the Service without removing himself from the professional resources essential to his practice of medicine. Some practitioners remained wholly outside, but most came in, and of these many expected that their practices would combine a reasonable proportion of private patients.[91]

The method of remunerating doctors at the start of the scheme encouraged general practitioners to have large Health Service practices. Doctors were paid a standard capitation fee and were permitted a large list of 4,000 National Health Service patients. In 1953, the system of payment was changed to favor smaller lists. A loading factor was added for patients between 500 and 1,500 and the maximum list for single practitioners was reduced by 500. Thus, a doctor with a list of 1,500 patients received an increase in remuneration from capitation of 43 per cent as contrasted to an increase of 20 per cent for a doctor with a maximum number of patients.[92] This principle of remuneration for smaller or medium sized lists continued in future awards, and even greater financial incentives were given for a "moderate size" list.[93] The size of list beyond the leading limits became a less and less important determinant of doctors' income. However, even so it was felt by the Pilkington Commission that list size was too influential, and the Commission recommended that more emphasis be placed on other items than capitation in fixing income.[94]

The Review Body's 1966 recommendations implemented this policy by reducing significantly the role of capitation payments. Existing loadings were dropped, but the capitation fee was increased for older patients, and special payments were introduced for doctors' work outside normal working hours, including additional fees for visits made between midnight and 7:00 A.M. Payment for out-of-hours work was to be further compensated by a supplementary capitation fee for all patients above 1,000 on the doctors' lists. In addition, special fees were provided for particular services, e.g., for cervical smears, vaccinations, immunizations. The Review Body recommended that expenditures on rents and rates for doctors' premises should be reimbursed, as well as 70 per cent of expenditure on ancillary help. A major innovation was the "basic practice allowance" to be paid to all doctors with a minimum list of 1,000 patients "available . . . within normal hours for certain minimum periods each week." This allowance would be supplemented for doctors having special qualifications and seniority, and for doctors practicing in unattractive areas and in groups. The basic allowance and its supplements would be lowered for those doctors who did not meet the minimum requirements of full practice.[95] The B.M.A. described the basic practice allowance as "the most satisfactory method of recognizing" that the practitioner has certain commitments in expenditure, time, and work which do not vary with the size of list.[96]

The earlier policy of loadings and the Pilkington Commission's introduction of the basic practice allowance, while in accord with the need for a better distribution of patients and reduced lists to ensure better medical attention for patients, at the same time made it possible for doctors to take maximum advantage of National Health Service remuneration and increase their earnings outside the Service. Under the loadings policy this was particularly true of partnerships where the average of the two lists rather

than the individual lists was calculated to obtain maximum loading remuneration. Thus, one doctor with a relatively small National Health Service list and a large private practice might enter
a partnership with a doctor with a large list. On average size, all
the Health Service patients in the 500 to 1,700 range for each doctor would be compensated for at the loading rate, although one
doctor might have two-thirds or more of the total patients on his
list. Under the 1966 Review Body's recommendations, the basic
list is 1,000 or an average of 1,000 for partnerships, and there is
a stipulation about the doctor being available for a minimal contractual working week. There will, no doubt, be some difficulty
in enforcing the latter.

The Pilkington Commission was not unaware of the participation of Health Service doctors in private practice. Its own survey
indicated that 10 per cent of Health Service general practitioners
saw private practice as their "main" activity while another 25 per
cent gave it as a "subsidiary" activity. Although the terms "main"
and "subsidiary" may be loosely interpreted, it could at least be
assumed that private practice involved a significant part of the
time of 35 per cent of general practitioners. The members of the
Commission showed their concern about the possibilities for
increasing private practice when questioning witnesses who
recommended the shortening of doctors' lists. As one member
of the Commission stated:

I am raising the question of the care of the patient. If the argument is that you care better for the patient under the Health Service by reducing the list, then it would *ipso facto* follow that if the
doctor would then enter into work outside the Health Service, the
argument falls to the ground.[97]

At another point in the hearings, a member of the Commission
asked:

Under these proposals before us you visualise that at a certain
stage a doctor who had 3,500 on his list would receive the same
salary when he dropped down to 2,000. Would you then suggest

he should have complete freedom to deal with his private patients? He would have lost 1,500 off his list, and he would suffer no reduction in his salary. Would you suggest that he should still go on with private patients without control?[98]

On the whole, the witnesses favoring the reduction of doctors' lists were vague about the principle of limiting the amount of private practice or the possibilities of establishing any practical procedures of control.[99]

Undoubtedly, the Commission and the Review Body were influenced by other considerations than the opportunities for private practice when they made their recommendations. Trends in private general practice did not show it to be an immediate danger to National Health Service practice. More critical was the fact that if doctors generally were dissatisfied with the terms of their contract there would be less incentive to enter or remain within the Service, a greater loss than the diversion of a small amount of doctors' energies into private practice. The terms of the 1966 Review Body's recommendations were made during the threat of mass resignations by the B.M.A. and the development of the B.M.A.'s scheme of insurance for private general practice. The annual subscription rate and the fees for service under this scheme were arranged to provide the doctor with a higher income than the Health Service's standard and supplementary capitation and out-of-hours fees for patients beyond the basic list of 1,000.

The disregard by the government of the doctors' engagement in private practice may have been the only realistic approach unless rigid standards and controls were introduced. Although general practitioners have complained bitterly about the size of their lists, there is no evidence, apart from those engaged wholly in private practice, that a large private practice necessarily signifies a relatively small list. The Report of the Pilkington Commission, for example, does not indicate whether practitioners who reported private practice as a "main" or "subsidiary" activity had fewer Health Service patients than other practitioners. The concept of private practitioner tends to be used relatively rather

than absolutely, and doctors or partnerships with a majority of
Health Service patients may be viewed and view themselves as
essentially in private practice because of the high proportion of
private patients compared to other practices. Among the small
sample of practices examined in this study there appeared to be
no clear relationship between the size of the two types of practice. For example, in the case of a single practitioner with over
3,000 patients, one-third of his active current cases were private
patients. A partnership practice of two physicians with almost
5,000 National Health Service patients received a quarter of its
income from private patients while in another partnership of
three full-time and one half-time physician with a total of 6,000
National Health Service patients, less than 10 per cent of income
came from private practice.

Although the amount of private practice which any doctor
might have was a matter for individual choice, the participation
of doctors in private practice affected the contract of all doctors
with the state. Until the recommendations of the Pilkington Commission in 1960, private earnings, earnings from private patients
and other private sources such as insurance and industrial companies, were assumed to be £2 million and were subtracted from
the total pool for doctors. Thus, the average income of all doctors
was reduced by the calculated gross private practice income. The
Pilkington Commission recommended that private earnings be
dropped from consideration in the pool because they were "very
difficult to ascertain on an exact or agreed basis" even though it
was recognized that no matter how small a doctor's list he added
a full unit to the total earnings for doctors under the pool.[100]

The exclusion of private earnings from the pool still left the
question of reimbursement for practice expenses. The government, in reimbursing general practitioners for their total practice
expenses, recognized that some of these expenses were incurred
for practice outside the National Health Service. The Review
Body, in 1966, maintained that it had now a more accurate estimate of income and expenditures in this type of practice and
recommended that these expenditures be disregarded when cal-

culating the government's reimbursement. In doing so, the Review Body noted that average levels of net income would probably have been higher in the past had not some allowance been made for the inclusion of expenses incurred in other than Health Service practice.[101]

The relationship of private to Health Service practice in the hospitals has been of an entirely different order. The private practice of the general practitioner, apart from such indirect effects as it might have on his Health Service practice, was unrelated to the Health Service. Private specialist practice was not only integrated within the hospital structure, but the right to this practice was defined by the nature of the hospital appointment. As the Report of the General Practitioners' Association stated in comparing the relative positions of the consultant and the general practitioner:

The consultant is free to seek and carry out private work in his specialty . . . unless he is whole-time.

He may provide a separate consulting room for this purpose. He is able to use the hospital facilities for private work, although these are charged to the patient over and above his professional fees. No capital or maintenance cost fall on the consultant for hospital facilities, including physical apparatus.[102]

Although private practice is, for all practical purposes, identified with the part-time consultant, even the whole-time consultant can do a limited amount of private practice. Like the part-time consultant, he may be paid for professional services outside the scope of the Hospital and Specialist Services under the Health Service. For example, reports on patients not under observation or treatment at the hospital, examinations and reports for prospective immigrants, and examinations and reports required for entrance to professional training or employment, may be arranged privately between those desiring the service and the consultant.[103] If hospital laboratory or radiological facilities are required, the fee charged represents payment for professional services and hospital costs. If such is the case, the hospital receives compensation; if not, the fees are entirely for professional services and belong to the consultant.[104]

For the part-time consultant to whom private practice has been a major source of income, the hospital's contribution of facilities was a necessary condition of his practice. However, from the start of the Health Service the position of the part-time consultant was additionally strengthened by conditions of service relatively more advantageous than his whole-time colleague. The Spens Committee set the tone of early policy by maintaining that

the responsibilities and commitments of a part-time appointment cannot be measured, in relationship to those of a whole-time appointment, simply by comparing the total working hours of the part-time officer with the total working hours of his full-time colleague. The specialist who holds a part-time hospital appointment has a continuous responsiblity for the patients in his charge, which must extend beyond the limits of the time he contracts to serve; further, he will be expected to take his share in the committee work of the hospital, and this must encroach upon time which would otherwise be spent in private practice. In assessing the remuneration which shall attach to part-time appointments such factors must be taken into account.[105]

With this in mind, the Spens Committee recommended that the part-time specialist be given additional compensation of 25 per cent over that of a whole-time specialist for the same period worked by the part-timer.[106] The government opposed the principle of weighting, and the Pilkington Commission recommended, in 1960, that no new appointment should include the weighting factor.[107] The Commission explicitly rejected the argument of the Spens Committee and pointed out that the responsibilities of part-time consultants did not differ from other staff who had a continuous responsibility for their patients and that committee work was shared by many persons who received no compensation whatsoever.[108]

In addition to the advantages of salary weighting and calculation of sessions, the part-time consultant, at the start, had a special or extra fee granted him for domiciliary consultations. Until November 1955, only part-time consultants were eligible for such fees at the basic rate of four guineas per consultation with a maximum of 800 guineas in one year. At that time, whole-time consultants also became entitled to remuneration similar to that of domiciliary consultants, except that the first eight consultations in any quarter had to be rendered free in view of their whole-time commitments.[109]

Although the specific terms of the contract of service gave the part-timer advantages which have been somewhat moderated in time, the part-timer, as compared to his whole-time colleague, received more generous treatment in other ways, particularly from the system of traveling expenses, distinction awards, and the estimation of income taxes. The Spens Committee provided for awards to part-time consultants who would engage in private as well as public practice with the rationale of attracting specialists into the public service. Their ideal of remuneration was a system of professional compensation which would make it unnecessary for the specialist in public service to turn to private practice to supplement his earnings.[110] However, as noted above, in its actual operation the award system has been greatly to the advantage of part-time consultants. Although it has been maintained by some that the part-timer is generally superior to the whole-timer and that his very ability to succeed in private practice is indicative of his pre-eminence, the differences in the proportions of awards would seem too great to be accounted for entirely in this fashion. Among the factors that stand out is the high proportion of awards given in specialties permitting a relatively large amount of private practice, particularly general medicine and general surgery, each with at least 50 per cent more awards than their proportion of the total number of consultants. On the other hand, specialists in physical medicine, radiology, and pathology, all of whom tend to be full-time consultants, received less than their appropriate share of awards.[111] Since the administration of awards is highly informal and secret, no official rationale has been offered for the differences in awards among specialties and between part-time and full-time consultants, and the awards may reflect the latent status of prestige structure within the profession more than any valid distribution of merit. The mechanics of selecting consultants for awards bears much resemblance to identifying the elite in relatively close social systems.[112]

The advantages of the part-time consultant in the total income obtained from both public and private sources have been further increased by the tax treatment of his income. Until 1961, when it was disallowed by a decision of the House of Lords, the part-time consultant had been able to include expenses incurred in his Health Service position as deductions from his private practice income.[113] Even with the 1961 limitation the part-time consultant can still claim many of the normal expenditures of professional life as practice expenses in contrast to his whole-time colleague who cannot maintain that his expenses are necessary for employment as defined by the tax officials.

The balance of part-time and whole-time consultants in the National Health Service has been influenced by the option given consultants to choose whether they prefer whole-time or maximum part-time service. Normally, a post has been thrown open to all who are interested in "substantially" full-time employment. After the candidate has been selected, he may then opt for either whole or maximum part-time practice. Similarly, after his appointment the consultant may choose to change his status from either one to the other, and the "circumstances and preferences" of the consultant are given heavy weight in any decision by the hospital.[114] In fact, there is a reasonable amount of switching by consultants as whole or maximum part-time positions fit them more satisfactorily at different points in their career. Consultants whose specialty draws a lucrative private practice will prefer maximum part-time during their years of highest productivity when they can carry the responsibilities of both Health Service and private practice. Later in their careers, they may prefer the relatively less taxing role of whole-time consultant while at the same time increasing their superannuation benefits from Health Service employment.

The supporters of part-time consultant service maintain that it attracts the most able to the public hospitals, it distributes specialist personnel to all regions, it gives consultants the benefit of outside experience, and it results in the Health Service's obtaining as much consultant effort, sometimes more economically, as when whole-time personnel are employed. On the other hand, it has been stated that the efficiency and morale of the services would be higher under a whole-time consultant service. An analysis of the comparative costs of whole-time and part-time consultants in the National Health Service in the mid-1950's indicated that the unit of part-time work was one-third higher if all factors, including tax advantages, were taken into account.[115]

In practice neither party, when in power, has encouraged the expansion of part-time posts. The gradual whittling away of the part-time consultants' advantages occurred while Conservative governments were in power. The Chairman of the B.M.A.'s Central Consultants and Specialists Committee remarked bitterly, "It was ironical that all these changes to the detriment of private practice had occurred under the rule of a Conservative Government, supported by a Party which had always alleged that it strongly supported the continuance of private practice."[116] There has been some justification for the complaints of junior hospital staffs and consultants in the early 1960's that the contracts for part-time consultants were less favorable and that young consultants were not as encouraged to look to private practice and part-time consultant posts.[117]

In 1966, the Ministry sought to reduce the discretion of the consultant in determining whether a post would be a whole-time or maximum part-time. The Minister attempted to clarify the confusion about the rights of hospital boards by emphasizing that if a board thought that a full-time post was needed, it could be advertised as such with no part-time option.[118] This had evidently been a sensitive issue in the administration of the Service. The Ministry's memorandum to the Pilkington Commission in 1957 recommended that hospitals be free to appoint whole-time consultants as necessary and expressed the hope that agreements could be worked out amicably in contrast to some of the conflict in the past.[119] With the strengthening of the hand of the boards and the possibly greater influence of whole-time consultants in the councils of the profession in the future, the maintenance of the role of the part-timer may become a less crucial issue.

Support for Private Practice

Although the National Health Service, as already noted, is a preponderantly public scheme with almost all of the citizenry obtaining their health benefits as full members, there is a small proportion of the population who, on the whole, make use of both the Health Service and private practice. Thus, even apart from the fact that practitioners of private medicine make a considerable part of their income from the National Health Service and that some private facilities like hospital care are provided by the public structure, the effectiveness of private medicine today depends on the general availability of public resources. The private patient of a general practitioner with or without a National Health Service list receives the full support of the public laboratory and out-patient facilities. While the private patient is denied drugs under the National Health Service, the cost of the services from his general practitioner is materially reduced by the resources which the doctor can obtain for him without charge.

There has, however, been a strong demand on the part of those interested in the expansion of the private sphere for greater government encouragement of private medical care. Some of the exponents of greater government support of private medicine are opposed to a universal service like the Health Service and would like to return to a basically private approach to medicine.[120] For them, more government support of private medicine is at best a temporary expedient or at worst a harsh compromise with current political realities. Although the private market is viewed as the most effective means of relating supply and demand, there is little likelihood of a speedy abandonment of the National Health Service, and the most practical approach, as viewed by its opponents, may be a combination of subsidies for those using the private sector and a reduction of benefits for those in the public program. While there has been much discussion in principle about the value of a totally free market in health and other services and the disadvantages of government involvement, current proposals for change assume a large and continuing role for government. Even from the Fellowship for Freedom in Medicine, the most consistent and energetic critic of the National Health Service, there have come suggestions merely for shift in balance between public and private expenditure, with a greater proportion of expenditure, some 25 per cent, coming from private sources.[121] This expansion of the private field, it is assumed however, is dependent on government encouragement, and the state's support must, therefore, be distributed across the whole of both public and private care.

During the years since 1948, several methods by which government might support the private provision of medical care have been suggested. Among the most regularly recommended has been tax relief for those purchasing their own private health insurance. The Fellowship for Freedom in Medicine has pressed for such a measure persistently,[122] and the provident societies have been actively interested in tax reductions for their subscribers. The Porritt Committee, in its report to the B.M.A., supported tax allowances for private schemes as the most "practical" approach. "Not only do the schemes provide an incentive for private practice," stated the Report, "but they also relieve the demands on the National Health Service and thus make a contribution towards the tasks of lessening overall Health Service costs."[123]

The government, whether Labour or Conservative, has given little encouragement to the advocates of tax allowances for those insuring privately. However, in fact, a significant proportion of current premium payment is tax allowable under corporate rather than individual tax regulations. Although an individual cannot claim a tax benefit for his premiums, the amount paid by the company can usually be charged against profits and is generally not considered to constitute income of the employee for tax purposes. In view of the growing adoption of schemes of private health insurance by companies for their employees, there is, at present, a considerable tax subsidy to the cost of private medical care.

Government grants to those choosing to opt out of the Health Service have also received some consideration. The B.M.A., in 1954, thoroughly reviewed the issues of opting out without paying a contribution to the general medical services and of grants-in-aid toward the cost of private nursing home treatment,[124] and concluded "reluctantly" that "neither of the propositions was in fact practicable."[125] The possibilities of either opting out or improving the Service were almost equally supported by the sample surveyed in 1965 by the Institute of Economic Affairs. Of the total, 34 per cent favored contracting out and paying less contributions while 32 per cent favored a heavier tax investment for improved health services for all. A small proportion of the sample, 25 per cent, favored limiting the state health services to the needy and thus, reducing the public cost.[126] The B.M.A. survey by the Porritt Committee showed little professional support for the right for patients to contract out, although the doctors did favor grants-in-aid for those using private care.[127]

The Institute of Economic Affairs survey had dealt with the issue of grants-in-aid through its questions on preferences for vouchers to pay partially for the cost of private health insurance. Apart from the complexity of the questions and of the choices offered respondents which affected the survey as a whole, the reliability of responses to the voucher questions was limited by the failure to make clear to the respondents the extent to which they would continue to be taxed for the National Health Service and what their total private costs might be. Thus, it is difficult to appraise the significance of the 23 and 30 per cent of the sample, who, under varying conditions, would choose the vouchers presumably in preference to the National Health Service.[128] In general, the Institute concluded that its findings pointed to strong support for the contracting out from the Health Service which could be governed by individual choice or by income standards of eligibility for the public service.[129]

This more limited role for the Health Service as well as for other social services has been advocated by those who oppose universal coverage and who maintain that the state should concentrate its efforts on the needy while the remainder of the population is free to make its own arrangements on the private market. This position is rationalized by the assumed affluence of contemporary society, and the resultant policy would have much resemblance to the state of affairs in the social services prior to the reforms following World War II. However, the effective provision of basic services is not entirely, or even significantly, influenced by the capacity or willingness of a minority to finance their own care, and the surveys thus far undertaken do not provide sufficiently valid indicators of the numbers who would prefer other forms of health coverage.

CHAPTER 5

Private Practice: The Doctors' Dilemma

THE resolution of the role of private practice under the National Health Service is affected by the three major components of the system of health care: the public, the state, and the medical profession. In the almost two decades since the start of the Health Service, the public and the state, as represented by government policy, have demonstrated a tolerant, but not encouraging attitude toward the presence of private practice. The public has shown a declining interest in private general practice while private specialist and hospital practice has, for the most part, maintained a relatively constant position among a limited segment of the population. Government policy, whether under Conservative or Labour control, although not firmly antagonistic to private practice, has resulted in a gradual diminution of opportunities and resources for the provision of private medical care. Under these circumstances, the existence of private practice has to a large extent depended on the medical profession itself. Although other interests, such as the large provident societies, are involved, their resources and public are minor in comparison with the state provision, and whatever success they may have will be primarily influenced by the continued identification of some significant segment of the medical profession with the practice of private medicine.

The medical profession, however, cannot in any sense be viewed as a unity in its reaction to private practice. The number of general practitioners with little or no private practice far exceeds those with any real attachment to private care. Although the number of part-time paid consultants is more than twice the number of whole-time paid consultants, the paid part-time staff make up less than 30 per cent of those in the various medical and dental professional grades of hospital staff.[1] Even among part-time consultants, there is a wide range in the extent of private practice.[2] The experience and attitudes of doctors before 1948 must also be taken into account. Specialists had been greatly oriented to the opportunities of private practice, and in negotiations at the start of the Health Service preferred to keep themselves free of a full-time commitment.[3] Many general practitioners, particularly in industrial areas, relied almost entirely on panel patients and their families. A smaller group had lucrative practices of upper class private patients, and it was these physicians who resented most bitterly the passing of private practice and the consequent loss of income when many of their former patients joined the National Health Service.[4] In time, this group of general practitioners has had a lessening influence among family doctors, whereas among consultants the tradition of private practice and the position of part-time specialists in the Health Service has had a continuing vitality.

Thus, there has been a major difference between consultants and general practitioners in their identification with private practice. In fact, the relative ease with which the consultant may engage in private practice and earn additional income has been a source of resentment among general practitioners. Prior to the Health Service, the consultant was dependent to a large extent on referrals from general practitioners. With the Health Service the consultant was greatly freed from his reliance on the family doctor for business,[5] and it has been suggested that private practice would encourage better relationships since consultants would be more conscious of practitioners if they were dependent on them for referrals.[6]

The advantages of private practice for the consultant have been further brought home to the general practitioner by the attitudes of some of their patients. Patients who do not want to pay general practitioners for the benefits of private care will, on entering the hospital, seek a pay-bed and a private consultant. Even if a general practitioner is permitted to visit one of his Health Service patients who is a private hospital patient, he is not permitted to charge a fee. However, most general practitioners do not have hospital privileges, and even for those who do there are few beds and even fewer for private patients.[7] At present, the only real source of private in-patient income for general practitioners would be from private patients in private hospitals and nursing homes, and these fees are not covered by the provident societies. At the start of the Health Service, there was some effort to gain for private general practitioners hospital privileges, but the government refused on the grounds that it had no intention of permitting doctors outside the Service to enlarge their practices at the expense of the Health Service hospitals.[8] The profession, or at least those concerned with private practice, have continued to press for the "right" of the general practitioner to treat his private patient in the hospital.[9]

However, the difference between the general practitioner and the consultant have not only been related to the immediate opportunities for private practice but also to the general advantages of the consultant under the National Health Service which are exacerbated by the private practice privileges. Thus, the relative exclusion of the general practitioner from the hospital service has widened the breach between the consultant and practitioner.[10] The expansion of general practitioner appointments to hospital staffs has been strongly recommended by recent governmental advisory committees concerned with the functioning of the family doctor in the National Health Service.[11] The general morale of the family doctor has received much attention, and it has not been improved by comparisons with the consultant and the impression given that the family doctor is an inferior journeyman while the specialist is a master craftsman.[12] From the time of the original negotiations of the government with the medical profession, the government made concessions to the consultants, including more status and financial rewards as well as opportunities for remunerative private practice, which have made the general practitioner sensitive to the favored position of the specialist and the conflict of interest between the two branches of the profession.[13]

Within general practice itself, the issue of private practice has been the source of some conflict. For aside from his possibly abstract sympathy with private practice, the family doctor primarily engaged in Health Service practice has had little to gain from the existence of private practice. Until the Pilkington Commission recommended in 1960 the removal of the calculation of private earnings from the pool for doctors' remuneration, the average compensation for all doctors was reduced by the estimated earnings of £2 million from private sources.[14] In the differences between the Ministry and the B.M.A. over the provision of drugs under the Health Service to private patients, the Minister of Health, in 1954 and 1956, reminded the profession that any increase in private practice income as a result of such action would result in a corresponding decrease in the government's contribution to the central pool for all practitioners.[15] The doctors identified with private practice felt that their interests were not being properly represented by the B.M.A.[16] This reaction was crystallized at the 1956 Annual Representative Meeting when those pressing for drugs for private patients criticized the leadership sharply for their failure to obtain this objective and succeeded in having a resolution passed for greater representation of those actually in private practice on committees negotiating with the Ministry on the question of drugs.[17]

The doubts of doctors with an interest in private practice that their demands were being strongly enough pressed were not entirely unwarranted. When the Private Practices Committee applied pressure for action on the drug proposal, the General Medical Service Committee, the B.M.A. committee responsible for representing general practioners in negotiations with the government, responded that although private practitioners would

only gain from it, Health Service practitioners could only lose
from it.[18] Again at the time of the 1965 negotiations, the Chairman of the General Medical Services Committee excluded the
question of drugs because he did not think it relevant to service
under the Health Service. In response to the objections of the
Chairman of the Private Practices Committee and others that the
negotiations were supposed to cover all matters affecting the
future of general practitioners and that private practice was essential to medicine, it was finally agreed that a separate communication would be sent to the Ministry on the matter of drugs for
private patients.[19] As a result of the 1965–66 negotiations, the
Review Body, as noted above, recommended a further reduction
in the effect of private practice on the income of practitioners.
The expenses of private practice had been included in the total
reimbursement allowed by the government for general practitioners. The Review Body noted that this had reduced the average net income fixed for all doctors, since larger amounts would
have been credited to the pool if it had not been assumed that
expenses unrelated to National Health Service general practice
were being provided for.[20]

Those concerned with the maintenance of private practice
wanted lists of private practitioners to be established and made
publicly available for patients seeking private attention. Again
they received little encouragement from the B.M.A., whose Ethics
Committee objected to a special list and indicated that the
General Medical Council of the Ministry of Health would not
approve of such a device for publicizing private practitioners.[21]
The frustration of the supporters of private practice was evidenced in the late 1950's when they objected that the Private
Practices Committee, heretofore the bulwark of their interests,
was not sufficiently representative of their needs, and a Private
Practice Group, solely concerned with private general practice,
was established within the B.M.A.[22] The Group, however, has not
been active or influential. The Fellowship for Freedom in Medicine has been continuously critical of what it believed to be the
insufficiently aggressive stance of the B.M.A. on private practice,

and during the 1965–66 negotiations other groups, such as the General Practitioner's Association and the Birmingham Action Group, independently pressed forward with the cause.

The differences among general practitioners about private practice have been more marked among consultants. The opportunities for friction are greater between part-time consultants engaging in private practice and whole-time consultants fully employed in National Health Service hospitals. The separate interests of the two are indicated by the existence of a Whole-time Consultants' Association to represent the full-time publicly employed clinicians. Consultants presented their evidence to the Pilkington Commission under the aegis of both this Association and the Joint Consultants' Committee. Although the latter officially represents both whole-time and part-time consultants in negotiations with the Ministry, its evidence showed a bias in favor of the part-time consultant in contrast to that offered by the Whole-time Association. Since the great majority of consultants are part-time and the profession is dominated by the most influential of these, it is not surprising that their interests should be stressed.

Some of the differences between the two types of consultants have arisen from what the whole-timers have considered the more advantageous terms of service afforded the part-timers in the National Health Service. However, in the opinion of part-timers this dissatisfaction is not warranted in view of what the Joint Consultants' Committee noted as "the advantage of a comparatively regular professional existence, free from the unpredictable stresses of private practice."[23] From the Committee's point of view, "the great disadvantage of the whole-time consultant's position is that he lacks the sense of professional independence that is felt by a consultant not wholly dependent on his salaried appointment."[24] And the Committee concluded that "private consulting practice makes a distinctive contribution to medicine which indirectly benefits the Health Service and is a means of attracting to medicine some of the most successful practitioners who, without opportunities for private practice, might well decide to seek their fortunes elsewhere."[25]

The whole-time consultants view less optimistically the compensations of private practice and particularly its contribution to the National Health Service. Although they have not questioned the assumption that part-time staff often do more than their contract calls for, they have pointed out that there are differences in the approach to their hospital responsibilities of part-time consultants who are developing a private practice and full-timers solely involved in hospital work. In effect, the burden of maintaining the hospital as a "going concern," according to the whole-timer, falls upon the full-time staff.[26] This not only affects the whole-time consultants, but also the junior staff, who may even be expected to look after the private hospital patients of the part-time consultants. Since the junior staff cannot charge for this service, they are dependent on the not always forthcoming generosity of the consultant.[27] It was suggested before the Guillebaud Committee that the presence of part-time consultants had led to a greater need for junior staff who could deputize for the consultant.[28]

These are, thus, objective and psychological sources of friction between the part-time consultants and the full-time hospital specialist staff. Since 1948, some of the more evident financial inequities for full-time consultants have been removed. There remain, however, possibilities for looseness in carrying responsibilities and for utilizing the hospital resources for private gain, which, although to a certain extent recognized perquisites of the part-timer, cause difficulties and resentment among those primarily identified with administering and serving the hospital system. These reactions are exacerbated by the tendency of some part-time consultants to emphasize their financial success and prestige.

Underlying the difference between those essentially in public practice and those relatively occupied with private practice, whether family doctor or consultant, are subtle factors of orientation and identification. At the beginning of the Service, the question was raised in Parliament of whether the tolerance within the National Health Service of practitioners undertaking both public and private practice would not destroy the confidence of the public in the whole scheme. Bevan replied that he had hoped as time went on this "dichotomy" would disappear.[29] Although to some extent this has happened, perhaps more striking has been the growing consciousness within the medical profession of the dichotomy.

The sense of difference has reflected some awareness on the part of doctors in the Health Service that the promotion of private practice, whether purposeful or not, has had strategic points of conflict with the development of a sound Health Service. The success of private practice has relied on the public's belief in its superiority and in the presence of important shortcomings in the National Health Service. In some services, such beliefs may have relatively minor consequences for the providers of the service and may mainly be the concern of the administrative bureaucracy. In a professional service like medicine, however, the implications are of primary significance to the professional staff. Doubts encouraged in the public reduce the morale and effectiveness of National Health Service doctors who, it is intimated, are practicing medicine of low quality. This is an attack on the professional ethic of doctors in the Service. Although all may not be its most ardent supporters, they consider themselves responsible professionals and, if they could not meet their idea of reasonable standards, they would not remain. As one doctor commented on the proposal for National Health Service drugs for private patients:

Why should I and my kind subsidise the private practitioner and his patients? It must be known to all that there exists a mistaken belief that the private practitioner is superior to the National Health Service doctor. Otherwise why would any patient pay for what he can get for nothing? This scheme will enhance that belief.[30]

Another doctor suggested that the public belief that it can get better medicine by paying for it privately is a "slur upon the medical profession."[31]

More serious for those identified with the Service and the reputation of the medical profession is the charge that inadequacies in the Service are used and sometimes created for the advantage of private practice. There has, for example, been much concern about "queue jumping" for hospital beds by private patients and even by Health Service patients who have arranged a private consultation or paid a domiciliary visit with a consultant.[32] Although recognizing that it happens, consultants generally voice disapproval at any priority given in regular National Health Service beds to patients who have seen the consultant privately.[33] On the other hand, there is some difference between many part-time consultants and the Ministry over the question of priorities for fully private patients, i.e., those using the hospital pay-beds. In January 1966, the Minister strongly criticized the possibility of people getting quicker treatment because they can pay.[34] For the private consultant, however, the matter of priorities is of great importance. In view of the frequently long waits for hospital attention, a major inducement for many private patients is the speed of getting into hospital or arrangements to suit one's own convenience,[35] and the consultant considers these to be rightful privileges of the private patient. Thus, it has been suggested that the part-time consultant has a vested interest in the long waiting period for hospital beds,[36] and that he may be little motivated to improve the conditions of National Health Service practice as long as he can gain from its inadequacies.

Although the Guillebaud Committee minimized the importance of queue jumping because of the few beds involved, the actual size of the problem has not been the major issue for critics within the profession. They are more concerned about the widespread rumors among the public which undermine faith in the administration of the Health Service and the ethics of the profession. One of the most virulent attacks on private irresponsibility in public medicine was made by *Lancet* in early 1961 when the question of queue jumping was attracting public attention. "To give priority to a patient," the editors wrote, "not because of clinical urgency but because he has paid a consultation fee, is not an exercise in professional freedom but more nearly an act of conspiracy."[37] The editors concluded with the warning that the profession might have to submit to rigid external controls if it did not use the discretion allowed it in the interests of the public. On the whole, the government has also preferred that the medical profession police its own conduct. Bevan, for example, while recognizing that some of the doctors were placing their private interests over the need for establishing a sound National Health Service practice, took the position that professional "disapproval" should be a major force in adjusting medical behaviour to the demands of the new Health Service.[38]

Bevan's views of the medical profession were often tempered by the practical problems of organizing a viable Health Service out of a reluctant profession. The doctors were particularly sensitive to losing their freedom in a state-administered service, and it may have been literally true, as one physician and Labour member of Parliament observed, that if it had not been for Bevan there would have been no opportunity for private practice in the Health Service.[39] On the other hand, it may have been well-nigh impossible to obtain the necessary cooperation of the doctors without such a concession. However, whatever Bevan's long-term views, his initial respect for professional autonomy has not proved ill-founded. Apart from the traditional shibboleths of the organizationally active leadership[40] (and even here there has been some change), there has been a noticeable ferment in doctors' attitudes and sense of professional ethic since the start of the Health Service. The demands of the new Service and its conflicts with earlier forms of medical practice have at least forced some reconsideration of previous conceptions of practice.

The concept of "inequality of consumption of medical care" may appeal to academicians and others impressed with the abstract advantages of a free market and even to some consultants and the few general practitioners identified with lucrative private practice.[41] For the great body of practitioners, however, the possibility of two standards of medicine is not an abstract issue for everyday practice. Since the rationale for private practice, when free medical care is available to all, must largely imply some service, the question of private practice cannot be comfortably divorced from the provision of two standards of care. The general practitioner has been more sensitive to the problem than the specialist because of the family doctor's traditional role of family counselor and his long-term relationship to his patients and their health needs. The "great man" image of the specialist may also make it easier for him to accept the notion of several rungs in the treatment hierarchy, roughly comparable to gradations in hospital staffing. Family doctors, on the other hand, have a more modest and uniform view of their talents.

The discomfort of the family doctor thus arises on several counts. If he has private patients, does he not have to provide them something more or different? Is this "something" a real product or dubious sales promotion? If it is real, does it mean that the Health Service patients he is also serving are getting less than the best he can offer? If so, is he comfortable with this situation? Some doctors say that they make clear from the start that they have nothing different to offer to private patients. For example, one doctor said, "Private patients are fools. They get no better treatment from me, often worse, because I hesitate about expensive drugs."[42] Other doctors will refer cynically to the snob satisfactions of the private patient as if this were sufficient reward to the patient for his payments.[43] Although such doctors may feel satisfied in not providing anything extra for the patient's fee, their attitude toward the private patient would not make for the best doctor-patient relationships. Moreover, at least among some physicians, there is uneasiness in accepting compensation when the patient is receiving nothing that he might not otherwise get under the Health Service. As one doctor who was not a strong supporter of the Service wrote in 1959 "In my experience, there are practically no patients who, after decent National Health Service attention, continue to hanker after private arrangements. . . . I am convinced that, in the main, large private lists will become an increasing reflection of the National Health Service doctor's attitude."[44]

Another group, and probably the largest having both Health

Service and private patients, say they offer the private patient something more but that this does not imply better medicine. Such doctors maintain that there is no necessary service denied their Health Service patients, but that they are willing to respond to the demands of private patients which they would refuse or discourage in Health Service patients. For example, a routine check for certain types of patients, which the doctor is confident can be adequately performed twice yearly, may be done at the request of a paying patient more frequently.[45]

The private patient would thus appear to obtain greater tolerance in terms of the time, the place, and the frequency of doctor contacts. "Some private patients are so," said one doctor, "because they like to feel they can send for you if they are just worried or anxious. It wouldn't be fair otherwise."[46] Other doctors, however, look less favorably on these requests. The amount of the doctor's time that he is willing, although not always called upon, to devote to the private patient is perhaps the most significant advantage of private care. Where ten minutes may be considered sufficient for a Health Service patient, a half hour or more may be allotted for a private consultation. Doctors interviewed in this study gave no reason to believe that the extra time resulted in better medicine, although the greater attention given the private patient may have had indirect consequences not always noted by the doctor. In general, the impression was given that the difference in time was devoted to establishing a more personalized and informal relationship with the patient. This, of course, can have a direct bearing on the patient's well-being. For example, as a consultant remarked before the Pilkington Commission, "The slight difference in the handling is that, to put it rather crudely, in an outpatients' session the patient listens to the doctor, whereas in a private practice the consultant listens to the patient."[47] It is difficult to appraise whether minimizing the significance of the greater time for the private patient represents a real evaluation or an unwillingness to recognize the possibly important differences in care given the two types of patient. In addition, the private patient can usually arrange appointments more to his own convenience and in his own home. The comfort and privacy of the patient are generally recognized perquisites of the private patient.

Against the complaints by doctors of the demands made upon them in the Health Service must be placed the willingness of some of those most critical of the Service to accept the greater demands of their private patients. Undoubtedly there are private patients who are even overconscientious in seeking to avoid making calls on the doctor's time. However, this is by no means true for all private patients, some of whom prefer the status of private patient for the very reason that they feel freer to expect more service.[48] The high incidence of such demanding private patients was a particular difficulty for the doctor-sponsored insurance schemes during 1966.

As already noted, many doctors do not encourage private practice, and a good number would not accept a patient privately. A major reason is unwillingness to view the patient as a customer and have a market relationship in their medical practice. Others, however, feel that if the patient pays for the service, he can make greater demands, and the demanding private patient is viewed differently from his Health Service counterpart. "One has sometimes been amused to hear how 'that neurotic worried about his heart' (under the National Health Service)," wrote a physician, "becomes 'this interesting case of a minor cardiac irregularity' (private)."[49] Another doctor with private patients said, "The doctor's attitude is slightly different with a private patient. You don't mind going around, when there's not much serious, compared with National Health Service when you do mind."[50]

Among some doctors the belief persists that payment for service is indicative of a valid health complaint on the part of the patient and a willingness to participate fully in treatment. Within the profession there has been continuous support for fee-for-service payment preferably with some direct contribution by the patient to the cost. Despite its reluctance, the leadership of the B.M.A. was pressed into including a fee-for-service proposal in its 1965–66 negotiations with the government,[51] and the Independent Medical Services scheme, the B.M.A. sponsored private medical insurance, incorporated a fee for service to supplement the patient's normal membership premium.

The resentment against what they considered over-use of their services was further exacerbated by the belief among some doctors that they could not rely on their own professional judgment to provide service without incurring the risk of government discipline should the patient complain. This was particularly true in the case of home visits at late hours which were a particular inconvenience to family doctors. With private patients they could do as they pleased, it was stated, whereas the possibility of having to answer the patient's charges before an official board made the public patient master in the doctor-patient relationship.

While the question of greater or less freedom in patient relationships is highly abstract, there has been nothing to indicate that the professional freedom of doctors has been threatened by the National Health Service, and the Service has usually been commended on its respect for professional rights.[52] A profession which previously had interpreted controls largely in its own interest would, however, feel that its partnership with government had some restrictive consequences. In 1965 the government further clarified the function of the general practitioner by advising patients that the decision about whether a visit to the patient's home was necessary was to be made by the doctor, who was "not under an obligation to see a patient whenever and wherever the patient thinks fit."[53]

While many doctors see little that they can give private patients in exchange for their fees and feel uneasy at encouraging an even unfounded notion of two standards of medicine, there are those who maintain that their private practice benefits their Health Service patients. According to these doctors, the idea of two standards is justified since the quality of care provided the private patient acts as a pace-setter for Health Service practice. Some doctors having both types of patient describe direct gains to their own Health Service patients by serving them with the additional equipment and improved facilities purchased from private income or considered necessary for private practice.[54] It is also maintained by these doctors that the doctor who limits his National Health Service practice prefers routine and seeks to avoid the more demanding and imaginative requirements of private practice.[55]

Whatever may be the effects of private practice on the Health Service, its existence has had interesting consequences for the nature of private practice. For doctors engaged in both types of practice, the financial security from their government income and super-annuation scheme has relieved them from too heavy reliance on the financial rewards of private practice. On the other hand, the income from private practice has become more certain since there is no reason for a patient who cannot pay remaining a private patient. In the past doctors felt ethically responsible for patients who could not afford care; under the Health Service such patients can join a panel and be assured adequate medical care. The Service is, in effect, a major medical insurance policy for the private patient. When the doctor or patient recognizes that the cost of treatment, as in the case of expensive drugs or hospital care, will be beyond the patient's means, the patient returns to the Health Service. In general, whether the grounds be personal or financial, the doctor need not be burdened with patients whom he does not want to treat privately when there is a readily accessible public system.

Thus, in some respects, the Service has simplified the administration of private practice. However, many doctors prefer to avoid mixing the two types of practice. They do not want to keep two sets of records and a separate appointment and billing system for private patients. With Health Service patients alone, they feel that they can plan their time more effectively for maximum professional services.[56] While the emphasis may be administrative, there is often an underlying discomfort in conciliating the demands of private practice with the needs of the Service and an appreciation of the extent to which doctors have been freed from the more onerous duties of earlier practice.[57] Although most general practitioners with private patients have panels, the ethical and administrative complexities of having both types of practice have led to the conclusion that the two types of practice are not wholly compatible. During the 1965–66 negotiations, those identified with the maintenance of private practice, such as some of the B.M.A. leadership and the Birmingham Action Group, insisted that general practitioners must choose either one form of practice or the other and that the mixture of the two was not a realistic alternative. One of the rationales offered for a fee-for-service system of payment was that it would remove the distinction between the private and the National Health Service patient since a standard fee could be charged for each item of service, and the only difference would be that the state would reimburse in the case of the latter.[58] The fee-for-service approach has been applied to the compensation of dentists, but it has not resulted in merging the two forms of practice as the fees and types of service offered have differed. Thus, the fee-for-service approach cannot be assumed to resolve the practitioner's difficulties with public and private practice.

Probably the most critical test of the general practitioner's view of private practice as a realistic alternative to the Health Service occurred during the conflict over doctors' remuneration during 1965 and 1966. In early 1965, the government's response to the profession's demands for increased compensation was an award of less than one-third of the total proposed by the doctors. The profession reacted sharply and quickly. A "Charter" was drawn up by the B.M.A. as the basis of any continued negotiations with the Ministry and a policy of withdrawal was approved. By April, over 17,000 doctors had filed their resignations with the B.M.A., and the outlines of an alternative private scheme were established.

The idea of withdrawal was not new. In 1950, the B.M.A. had devised the British Medical Guild as its parallel body for "collective action in disputes with public or other bodies."[59] At that time, the B.M.A. and its membership had entertained the possibility of a withdrawal from the Service in their negotiations with the government. Again, dissatisfaction with the government's remuneration policies in 1966 and 1967 resulted in serious consideration of resignation.[60] On both these occasions, however, despite strong support for withdrawal among some of the profession, the B.M.A. had not taken the preliminary step of collecting the resignations of doctors.

The issue of withdrawal in itself did not necessarily reflect a choice between the Health Service and any other form of practice. The resignations might at most be viewed as a strategic weapon to impress the government with the seriousness of the profession's demands. The threat of withdrawal thus might symbolize the profession's strong feeling of injustice and its willingness to back the B.M.A. fully in negotiating a better contract within the Service. There was much doubt about how many of those whose resignations were in the hands of the B.M.A. would actually leave the Service if the withdrawal policy were placed in operation. If response to the Independent Medical Scheme, the B.M.A.'s alternative to the National Health Service during withdrawal, may be considered as indicative of their intentions, only a relatively small proportion of doctors were seriously planning resignation. There was much pressure within the profession to support the idea of resignation, and many doctors probably forwarded undated resignations as evidence of solidarity with their colleagues.[61] As noted in the 1957 crisis, doctors favored the notion of withdrawal, but not for themselves.[62]

Support for withdrawal, however, was not limited to those who viewed it only as a strategy in negotiation. Among some, the crisis of 1965–66 and the reaction of the profession appeared to offer the testing ground for rejection of the Health Service and a return to private practice. For those antagonistic to the Service, here was the critical opportunity for launching an alternative service to compete with, and possibly in time replace, the existing one. The profession and the B.M.A. were pressed on all sides to take a strong stand. The Fellowship for Freedom in Medicine renewed its demands for greater encouragement of what its chairman called "highly subsidised Private Practice."[63] "Ideally everyone" would be "a private patient and not a panel patient."[64] The Fellowship believed that the B.M.A. tactics towards the Ministry were far too conciliatory, and while the term "Doctors' Strike" was not palatable, the Fellowship was irritated at the B.M.A.'s reluctance to bring about a withdrawal from the Health Service.[65] As the Fellowship became further disillusioned with the B.M.A. leadership, it concluded that "the one bright feature" was the Independent Medical Services. In the Fellowship's opinion, this was no "stop-gap measure, a useful weapon in negotiation, but a properly based proposal which carries the promise of a remedy for many of the ills of general practice today."[66]

However, the Fellowship's position was predictable, and its influence was limited to its declining membership of old guard opposition to the introduction of a state Health Service. More representative of segments of contemporary medical opinion was the Medical Practitioners' Union, with a membership of some 5,000 and affiliated to the Trade Union Congress and the General Practitioners' Association, an independent body with almost 3,000 members. The M.P.U. saw withdrawal as an appropriate measure to show the profession's dissatisfaction with the government's terms, but had little tolerance for those doctors who saw their "primary role as that of private contractors."[67] The G.P.A., on the other hand, heavily in favor of mass resignation, did not see the doctor as solely or essentially a participant in a state service. Founded in 1963, the G.P.A. maintained that family doctors suffered serious disadvantages under the National Health Service and that their interests had not been properly represented by existing organizations, particularly the B.M.A. The G.P.A.'s ideal of practice was the independent practitioner, and it was highly critical of the B.M.A.'s failure to support this goal. On its part, the G.P.A. marketed nationally its own private general practice insurance, the Family Care Service Ltd., some months before the B.M.A.'s scheme and before the completion of negotiations with the government. The cause of private practice was, however, most dramatically presented by thirteen doctors in Birmingham, the Birmingham Action Group, who resigned from the Service in the autumn of 1965 to enter private practice. For them, there was no alternative but to abandon entirely the National Health Service.

They had faith neither in the B.M.A. leadership nor in the possibility of the existing Service's being reformed to satisfy their expectations.

The demands for a more uncompromising position by the B.M.A. were not entirely limited to those outside the B.M.A. or those relying primarily on other organizations to effect their goals. Within the B.M.A. was reflected the struggle between those who saw the Health Service as the established and essential core of family medicine, whatever its limitations, and those who sought both to reform the Service to resemble more closely private practice and to increase the possibilities for independent medical practice. This conflict was evidenced in differences over the terms of the Charter, the use of the resignations, and the function of the Independent Medical Services.

The issue of payment by item-of-service has already been discussed. Although there had been great support for this method, including direct patient payment, in the Annual Representative Meetings just before and during the negotiations, the Charter gave small attention to the matter,[68] and in its negotiations the B.M.A. accepted the government's opposition to any serious consideration of fee-for-service as an alternate form of compensation.[69] Significant, too, was the statement included in the Charter that another alternative to the capitation fee was payment by salary, which although favored by "a smaller number" deserved consideration equally with the other methods. Official recognition by the B.M.A. of salaried compensation was a strong diet for those who equated salaries for doctors with the abolition of the kind of medical practice they valued.

The proposals in the Charter, whatever the acceptability of a salaried service, indicated that the medical profession, in the view of the B.M.A. leadership, was wholly involved in a government service and that the general practitioner, viewed abstractly, could not be seen as an independent contractor. A fundamental premise of the Charter was the establishment of a "reasonable" working period, and the suggested 5½ day week of 46 weeks pointed to a full-time contractual obligation. Additional payments were proposed for "over-time," i.e., night work and weekend consultation. It was also recommended that the state share, in addition to normal practice expenses, the cost of ancillary staff and the provision of improved premises and equipment. The partnership was to be so close that it would resemble the conditions which might prevail if the doctors were employed staff. Ideologically, however, the B.M.A. and its leadership were not entirely comfortable with this role for the general practitioner. In a special conference of representatives of Local Medical Committees to discuss the terms of the negotiations, the suggestion was made that the general practitioners' service be recognized as a whole-time occupation," and that doctors should get sufficient income so as not to need to subsidize their income from other work. There was some uneasiness among the representatives, however, about giving up the privilege of private and other types of practice, and the Chairman of the General Medical Services Committee, the responsible committee in negotiations, was strongly opposed to the general practitioner service being viewed as a whole-time commitment.[70] Yet the Charter and the negotiations with the Ministry made no reference to other forms of practice in which family doctors might be engaged, and the goal was clearly to establish a set of conditions for general practitioner service, including fees for special services and out-of-hours-work, which would meet practitioners' objections to the Health Service and reduce their incentives for other practice.

Although the Charter of the B.M.A. and its negotiations were the source of much dissatisfaction to those who wanted a harder line with the Ministry, the file of doctors' resignations was causing uneasiness and embarrassment to the B.M.A. leadership. Pressed into publicly taking an aggressive stance, they sought quietly to dispose of the resignations which constituted a latent threat to the continuation of negotiations. As long as the resignations remained potentially active, they distracted the membership's attention and support from the goal of reaching a feasible agreement with the government, and this, from the leadership's point of view, was the only practical solution. As the *British Medical Journal* advised the membership:

And at the end of it all doctors working in the National Health Service must face the uncomfortable fact that they cannot dictate their own terms, that they cannot themselves decide what their value to the community is. . . .

The Health Service is really still in an experimental stage, and everyone connected with it will have to exercise a good deal of patience and still more skill in devising different ways and means of bringing the experiment to a successful conclusion. And the success of the conclusion will depend upon the intrepretation the Review Body and Government—and the medical profession—make of the term of the National Interest.[71]

As soon as the Minister of Health made clear his intentions to evaluate seriously the demands of the profession, the General Medical Services Committee sought to dispose of the resignations. At the end of March 1965, a special representative meeting of the B.M.A. and a conference of delegates of the Local Medical Committees supported continued negotiations by voting to hold up the use of the doctors' resignations until June 30.[72] At the end of June, another delaying resolution, but with no time limit requiring reconsideration, was passed.[73] While a formal revoking of the resignations, as some of the leadership desired, seemed no doubt too great a loss of face to many of the profession, the delay had the same effect as initial enthusiasm wore off, and the doubts about the wisdom of withdrawal, always present in the minds of most doctors, became increasingly strong.

These doubts were reinforced by the recognition that, for most doctors, a state Health Service represented the most satisfactory form of medical practice. On the practical side, there was the realization that the public, as a Gallup Poll in February 1965, indicated, might be sympathetic to the doctors' plight, but would not approve of their resignation.[74] As early as 1950, one doctor had noted that the shift in the balance of income now coming from public sources has made anachronistic assumptions about the possibility of withdrawal based on earlier periods when doctors still had sources of private practice.[75]

Undoubtedly the public reaction to a strike by doctors, the general popularity of the Service, and the concern about serving their own patients as well as such considerations as income and other security benefits influenced the attitudes of doctors toward withdrawal. However, equally significant, although less tangible, was the family doctors' professional identification with the Service and the absence of any alternative, which, in their opinion, offered similar practical and professional advantages. As one doctor highly critical of the Service commented:

Most general practitioners whom I know are far more interested in practicing medicine, and being able to practice it properly, than having a direct confrontation with the Minister, disrupting the Health Service, and being forced to adopt a B.M.A. scheme of private practice which would appear to be a little more than a "pipe dream." To the individual G.P. mass resignation . . . spells potential financial disaster.[76]

It was clear from the start of the 1965 dispute that any proposal for withdrawal of general practitioners, no matter how vague, must be complemented by some alternative scheme of organized medicine. Since 1948 the whole of the profession and the public, and a large number before, had become accustomed to a culture of medicine far removed from the direct market relationship between physician and patient. Withdrawal from the National Health Service followed by individual private practice was inconceivable to the profession. The B.M.A. proposed to make feasible the resignation of its members by providing an insurance scheme for general practice. Independent Medical Services would substitute for the National Health Service and give some financial security to doctors. The Private Practices Committee and its chairman, Dr. Ivor Jones, moved ahead with the planning of the B.M.A. new insurance for general practice. Progress, however, was slow, and there was some concern in the Council of the B.M.A. as late as October 1965 that resignations might take effect before Independent Medical Services was in operation.[77]

Although some of the delay in establishing the insurance was a result of planning and administrative differences and difficulties, the major obstacle was the lack of interest of the B.M.A. membership. A questionnaire sent to general practitioners in the early months of 1965 indicated that a majority would use the scheme under any circumstances and that almost all would join if there were a mass resignation and would in any case voluntarily subscribe the £10 necessary for the capital fund to launch the project.[78] By October, only 4,200 of the 23,000 possible members had subscribed, and by the end of the year, 5,500,[79] with very few contributing after that time.[80]

The response of the family doctors to the Independent Medical Services was exceedingly disappointing to its advocates. The flush of support in the early poll suggested that the I.M.S. was linked, in doctors' minds, with their expectation of resignation. As they welcomed the B.M.A.'s negotiating with the Ministry and as their enthusiasm for withdrawal waned sharply, their interest in the I.M.S. as an alternative emergency protection also dropped. Within the Private Practices Committee, where concern for the insurance was centered, the small subscription fund was explained by some as confirming the general "meanness" of doctors toward spending money. Others, however, questioned the realism of the venture and even wondered whether the B.M.A. scheme might not have deleterious consequences for existing private practice.[81]

The £55,000 collected by the end of 1965 and the £57,000 by the summer of 1966, when the insurance was finally marketed, were far short of the minimal goal of £80,000 and the £200,000 desired to make the scheme fully operative.[82] More important than the actual shortage of capital was the clear evidence that few doctors would employ the scheme in their practices. Of the 25 per cent of general practitioners who contributed to the initial fund, how many could be counted on to introduce the insurance to their patients? Even the poll at the start of the negotiations, when enthusiasm was highest, showed a large difference between those who would subscribe to the necessary capital and those who would use the scheme.[83]

The indifference of the great majority of practitioners to a private insurance scheme and the evident relationship of the scheme with the plan for withdrawal, which no longer seemed at all likely, made for reconsideration of the projected insurance. The advocates of private practice, however, were determined not to lose the advantage of the B.M.A. sponsoring a general practice insurance. Dr. Ivor Jones pointed out to some of the doubtful members of the Private Practices Committee that, whatever the outcome of the negotiations, the Independent Medical Services would be continued, as "it was B.M.A. policy that there should be private practice for patients who preferred it." He also stressed the independence of the insurance from the issue of resignation.[84] In April 1966, a further appeal for support was made to the membership on the grounds that the insurance would enable doctors and patients who desired it to have private practice and that the practice thus encouraged would provide a "yardstick" for judging the state service and would help overcome "the dangers inherent in a State monopoly of medical practice."[85] The urgency of the scheme was, however, not broadly embraced. At the end of April, the Chairman of the Council, the representative executive body of the Association, drew attention to the resolution of one of the divisions to support the I.M.S. only if it were associated with mass withdrawal. Dr. Jones again pointed to the charge he and his committee had been given of establishing an insurance unrelated to the success of the negotiations.[86] It was apparent that a large group of influential B.M.A. leaders would have preferred quietly to drop the scheme, but the insurance's supporters were in no mood to compromise. The Independent Medical Services Ltd. was then established as an independent corporation. It was felt that although the schemes should have the "advantage of B.M.A. sponsorship," it "should have as few formal ties with the B.M.A. as possible in order to reduce the moral liability which the B.M.A. might otherwise be thought to bear."[87] While this might

be interpreted as a typical formal arrangement, it signified as
well the opposition of many of the B.M.A. leadership and their
desire to be as loosely connected as possible with the scheme.
The Independent Medical Services went into operation on
July 1, 1966. Although it was improbable that any doctors would
resign from the Health Service to practice entirely under the
I.M.S. the booklet prepared for doctors assured them that there
would be a "gross income sufficient to provide an adequately
staffed and equipped establishment without any need to either
unreasonably limit net income or attempt to look after a greater
number of patients than is compatible with the highest standards
of practice."[88] The sensitive issue of patient support was touched
upon by reference to surveys which, it was maintained, demonstrated that "some 30–40 per cent of the community would prefer to make private arrangements with their family doctor."[89]

The scheme provided general practitioner medical attention
and drugs at a monthly subscription rate with an additional
charge for patients living some distance from the doctor's surgery
and an item-of-service payment for each consultation according
to the place and time. The basic monthly subscription rate was
13s. for each adult, with a reduced charge of 8s. for the aged and
for young dependents. The mileage payments for patients over
two miles from the surgery made an additional monthly payment
of 1s. or 2s. depending on the distance. The service charges were
2s. 6d. for a surgery consultation and 5s. and 10s. for domiciliary
visits. The higher fee applied to night, week-end, or public holi-
day visits. Patients preferring to continue their present private
fee arrangements with doctors could limit their coverage to drugs
at a subscription of £1 1s. quarterly.[90]

The final terms of the scheme were the result of a series of com-
promises reached during the year of its planning. At no time were
the advocates of I.M.S. unaware of the difficulties of competing
with the Health Service. Despite the belief on the part of many
members of the B.M.A., and particularly those favoring private
practice, that some fee-for-service payment by the patient was
essential to good medical practice, the original plan omitted any

direct charge, and in effect, the subscription charge or "insurance contribution" as it was termed, bore a striking resemblance to the capitation fee under the Health Service. The Chairman of the Private Practices Committee in response to criticism explained that he had been advised that if the I.M.S. was to be viable it could not incur the antagonism of the public by a fee system. It was agreed that any charges beyond the subscription rate would depend on the discretion of the individual doctor.[91] However, when the scheme was launched a standard fee-for-service was an essential part. The charge to old age pensioners created further difficulties. On the one side, the aged, because of their medical needs, were more costly to treat, but, on the other hand, it was recognized that a high rate for the aged would be extremely bad publicity. The rate for the aged was fixed at a little more than 60 per cent of that for other adults.

The population to be covered was another subject of concern. A small doctor-sponsored scheme in the South-East had been selective of its patients. The practitioners had followed the policy of avoiding the bad risks and had advised the chronic sick to remain in the Health Service. The B.M.A. decided that it would have to offer a scheme to the total community, and let the patient make the choice between the I.M.S. and the Health Service. However, even the extent of the population to be covered by the projected insurance required careful consideration. The number of doctors who had made voluntary contributions to the capital fund did not indicate that the scheme would have widespread support in the medical profession. Some thought was given to limiting the operations of the insurance to three pilot areas, Yorkshire, Essex, and Birmingham, but it was decided that the scheme should honor its commitment to all doctors nationally who had shown an interest through their voluntary contribution and thus function on a national scale.[92] By the start of the scheme in July 1966, only 300 general practitioners had agreed to practice under the I.M.S.[93]

Although the General Practitioners' Association started its scheme several months before the B.M.A., there were no indications that it had made any real advance in attracting patients or doctors.[94] In general, the two schemes were similar except in regard to old age pensioners. The Family Care Service of the G.P.A. made no allowance for pensioners, and suggested that they "might prefer to remain under the National Health Service." In addition, although the F.C.S. was not limited to members of the G.P.A., it might have benefited from the better risks of the G.P.A. members' practices as compared to the broader population covered by the B.M.A. membership.

The major difference between the B.M.A. scheme and other attempts to insure general practice, whether commercial or doctor-sponsored, was the agreement reached with the pharmaceutical industry. The complexity of covering drugs' costs had convinced B.U.P.A. to exclude drugs from its plan. The Family Care Service and the doctors in the Birmingham Action Group had covered drugs in their subscription charges since no private scheme could hope to succeed if patients had to pay directly for drugs while there was no charge in the Health Service. On the other hand, the cost of drugs might raise the basic subscription charge beyond what the market could bear. The Family Care Service recommended, and the Birmingham doctors followed, the practice of bulk purchasing with as much doctor-dispensing as possible. This, however, was contrary to the interests of the local pharmacists who brought pressure on wholesale drug dealers supplying dispensing practitioners. Under the I.M.S. agreement with the Pharmaceutical Society, prescriptions for I.M.S. patients would be at the Health Service rate with an additional shilling for administrative expenses. The I.M.S. would guarantee the payment of all pharmacists' accounts.[96]

Although the I.M.S. leaders privately maintained that doctors must choose between being wholly within or wholly outside the Health Service, it was to be expected that doctors joining I.M.S. would continue their ordinary practice. The G.P.A. made it clear that doctors joining its scheme could continue to treat patients under the Health Service and that the Family Care Service could "exist alongside the National Health Service gradually evolving, and in some practices superseding it."[97] The real test, however, of the possibilities of private practice in contemporary Britain was the experience of thirteen Birmingham doctors and a scattered few in other communities who resigned from the Service during the 1965–66 negotiations to indicate their complete disillusionment with National Health Service practice. The circumstances were, on the whole, favorable. The medical community and much of the public were sympathetic, and Birmingham as an undoctored area provided more favorable conditions than other communities. The resigned doctors were, of course, affected by the Ministry's response to the situation, which was to provide, as quickly as possible, substitute medical attention. In Birmingham, the Minister guaranteed an adequate net income for three years to doctors filling the vacated posts because these doctors could not be sure of full lists nor the consequences to their practices if the resigned doctors returned to the Service.[98] The Local Medical Committee of Birmingham showed its support for the resignations by attacking the Minister's action in appointing replacements with a guaranteed income or "special financial inducement."[99] The issue was raised in Parliament of the poor treatment the new doctors were receiving at the hands of some of their Birmingham colleagues.[100]

The scheme of the Birmingham doctors, adopted by a few other doctors who individually left the Service, was in most respects the forerunner of the later G.P.A. and B.M.A. insurance schemes. Medical attention and drugs were covered. The subscription rates were somewhat lower than the Associations' schemes, but there was no reduction for the aged as in the I.M.S. Subscriptions, rather than being paid to the sponsoring organizations, which remitted them to the doctor less an administrative charge, were paid directly to the doctors. The Birmingham doctors estimated that their weekly net income per 1,000 patients under the scheme would be £59 as compared to £25 gross income under the Health Service.[101] Thus, they would be able to obtain a good income without the pressures of the normal patient load.

The actual practice experience of the doctors did not, however, fulfill their expectations on resigning. Few were able to maintain enough patients to make a reasonable income, and some doctors retained very few of their former patients.[102] For most patients, the medical attention under the Health Service was sufficiently satisfactory for them to be unwilling to be private patients of their former doctors in preference to being transferred to the list of another practitioner. Some patients could not afford the charges, and the National Assistance Board did not make grants towards private medical costs. Those patients who were drawn to the doctors in private practice often tended to be poor risks. The Birmingham doctors had attempted to weed out the chronically ill and most demanding,[103] but there were greater possibilities of having more such patients than was the case in the typical Health Service practice. In addition to the extra time required for such patients, they often incurred larger than average drug bills. Most of the resigned doctors were forced to accept other kinds of professional employment to supplement the reduced income from their own practices. Thus, it is unlikely that they achieved the leisurely conditions which they considered imperative for proper medical practice.

The limited success of the Birmingham doctors in their own practices was further exacerbated by their lack of support within the profession. Although they had assured the B.M.A. that they were not stimulating a movement toward private practice, they did see themselves as pioneers in totally rejecting Health Service practice. A Medical Practice Freedom Fund was set up to help resigning doctors so that their courage and sacrifices would be appreciated and have constructive consequences.[104] Although at the time of their resignations, they received much publicity and sections of the profession evinced interest and gave moral support, few doctors followed their example. Their success, even on a local level, depended on enough resignations so that patients might have to use private practitioners rather than rely on the overloaded practices of doctors remaining in the national scheme. The Minister could quickly replace a small number of resigning physicians, but this would not be feasible with a large withdrawal from the Service. However, the resignations expected by the Birmingham Group did not take place.[105] Most doctors preferred to view the Birmingham doctors' solution as unrealistic and unrelated to the major goal of reforming rather than defeating the National Health Service.[106] The experience of the Birmingham Action Group doctors gave little encouragement to those who looked forward to the attack of private practice on the stronghold of "state" medicine.

CHAPTER 6

The Future for Private Practice

SINCE the beginning of the National Health Service, radical changes have occurred in the practice of medicine. The organizational and technical evolution of medicine in Britain and elsewhere has made irrelevant some of the issues that were most salient and sensitive at the start of the Service. In the two decades since 1948, the concept then prevalent of the doctor as an independent contractor and private entrepreneur has retained at most a shadow-like reflection of its former meaning. Significant is the fact that in contemporary Britain only segments of the relatively young and old among general practitioners have demonstrated any active attachment to the idea of private practice. The General Practitioners' Association and the Birmingham Action Group consist primarily of young doctors who, having had no contact with private practice in the years before 1948, have on faith identified its image with all the goals of the medical profession. On the other side, the Fellowship for Freedom in Medicine has represented the hard core of those who opposed the Health Service from the start. More significant from a medical resource point of view than the opposition groups within the country have been the relatively large numbers of doctors who have been emigrating from the United Kingdom.[1] Although a variety of factors may account for this phenomenon, some of the mobility may reflect opposition to a public medical service and a desire to practice in an environment fully oriented to the income advantages of private medicine.

For most general practitioners, however, private practice presents ethical, technical, and administrative problems which they would prefer to avoid. Even among consultants, there has been noted some decline in interest in private practice.[2] As Sir Robert Platt has remarked of young consultants:

Although private practice can still be rewarding both financially and in experience, the young man of today does not particularly seek it, and often does not want it. His first aim is a good hospital appointment preferably with opportunities for research and training.[3]

While the issue of private medicine, for some, revolves around an ideological dispute about the appropriateness of the market system for supplying medical care as a private commodity, this is no longer too relevant in establishing the nature of medical provision. Except for a small minority, the profession does not today in Britain identify professional performance with independent and private medicine. Whatever the abstract values of medicine as a private enterprise, its realization would conflict radically with the profession's view of itself and its function.

As the reaction of general practitioners indicated, private practice involves a combination of administrative difficulties and emotional discomfort. As the problem of private practice for the consultant was summed up in *Lancet*, the private patient raises questions about the genuineness of medical practice. Patients who pay often come without the knowledge or approval of their family doctor. Desiring to avoid out-patient queues and seeking an early appointment, the private patient subjects the doctor to "barely disguised bribery." The doctor dislikes being "bought" and "dancing attendance on folk for what I can get out of them." The role of businessman is distasteful, and the rationale for private practice, that it results in a higher standard of medicine for all, is not justified.[4] Although some physicians may feel comfortable with the idea of two standards of medicine, the creation and maintenance of two standards are objectionable to many, and except for the cynical, the exploitation of the private patient without any real difference in service smacks of fraud.

There are in Britain a small number of family doctors who, for individual reasons or because of the nature of their practice, prefer to function as private practitioners. The Service has always permitted the general practitioner, and to a large extent the consultant, to determine the extent of his involvement. The 1966 contract was liberal in setting a list of 1,000 National Health Service patients as the requirement for the basic practice allowance for whole-time service. This would still allow the doctor much time for other types of practice. However, the need for strong inducements to engage in the Health Service is no longer a pressing problem. Private practice makes competing claims relatively weak in view of the general trends since 1948 and the little enthusiasm shown for it during the critical negotiations of 1965–66.

It is possible that this period may represent the last time when the profession as a whole gave serious consideration to private practice as an alternative to the Health Service. This is not to suggest that there is necessarily widespread approval of the functioning of the Service among physicians, but that conflicts will center around such other points of reference as the prestige and remuneration of various types of practice rather than the relative values of public and private medicine. The complaints of doctors are concentrated on bringing about advantages and reforms within the Service, not its abandonment. The lack of support for such attempts to revive private practice as I.M.S. and the Birmingham Action Group indicated that most physicians preferred to accept the broad outlines of the Service and press for changes within it.

Although the general practitioners' reaction to the Service has been influenced by remuneration, responsibilities, and terms of service, much of their feeling has been related to the vaguer, but probably more significant and universal problem of the role of the general practitioner in the field of medicine.[5] The frustrations, which are frequently voiced as antagonisms to the Health Service, are in fact the response of family doctors to a situation of ill-defined professional status and function.[6] Thus the conflicts within the Service must be seen as encompassing, as well as routine dissatisfactions, the resolution of the strategic and long-term problems of professional service whatever the immediate administrative environment. This dual nature of the relationship between the Service and doctors was noted in the B.M.A.'s final report to its members about its negotiations with the government on the "Charter for the Family Doctor Service." The negotiations, though primarily concerned with doctors' remuneration, covered a wide range of issues including the complex problem of the family doctor's relationship to the hospital service. The role of general practice within the total system of medical care remains of dominant concern. The organization of the National Health Service in 1948 did not resolve the complex problem of the function of the general practitioner and his relationship to the specialist and hospital system. This question is fundamental to medical practice everywhere, but concern for its solution has probably been intensified in the United Kingdom where the National Health Service has resulted in great emphasis on the economical and efficient use of medical resources.[7]

As differences within the service are worked out, there is an increasing probability that the Health Service or its equivalent will be viewed, as private medicine had been, as most conducive to the practice of quality medicine. For many doctors the solution to contemporary problems of better medical service has been identified with the potentialities offered by the new state system. To some extent this has been reflected in the greater willingness among general practitioners to consider the question of a salaried service. Several of the divisions of the B.M.A. showed interest in the introduction of salaries for general practitioners already present among consultants.[8] A survey of opinions of family doctors throughout the country by the B.M.A. late in 1964 concluded that "the family doctor has always insisted upon retaining the status of an independent contractor," but noted that a "minority" were giving support to a full-time salaried service.[9] The Charter included salary as one of the methods of remuneration to be negotiated. The radical nature of these proposals can be appreciated when it is recalled, as the Minister of Health pointed out, that doctors were so fearful of and opposed to a salaried service at the start of the Service that Bevan had felt compelled to reassure them by a statutory prohibition.[10]

The role of the B.M.A. is also indicative of the dominant attitudes within the profession as well as the function chosen for itself by the Association. Attacked by some as playing into the Ministry's hands and by others as being controlled by the most ardent advocates of private practice, the Association steered a course during the 1965–66 negotiations which, although releasing the energies of those most opposed to the Health Service, moved toward reaching agreement with the government. The doctors most actively engaged in the politics of the Association have generally been the most conservative. In view of the small number of B.M.A. members in private practice, the attention given the Private Practices Committee and the number of motions affecting private practice discussed and passed at the Annual Representatives Meeting (in 1965, 30 motions dealing with 15 matters)[11] were evidence of the political influence and pressure of those identified with private practice. The supporters of private practice were particularly active in 1965–66 as it was felt that the possibilities of any significant return to private practice in Britain were diminishing rapidly. Neither the Conservatives nor the Labour Party had been more than indifferent to the interests of private practice, and the dominance of the Labour Party in national politics spelled increasingly lean chances.

The B.M.A. continued its public espousal of the cause of private practice as it had almost yearly since 1948. It sponsored a policy of withdrawal from the service and the initiation of an independent medical insurance. Neither of these ideas originated with the B.M.A., and their adoption was tactically necessary if the Association was to maintain the support of the vast majority of general practitioners. However, through the B.M.A.'s reluctance to use the resignations, the enthusiasm for this action was gradually dissipated in the profession. The unwillingness to press for withdrawal and open criticism of groups such as the doctors of Birmingham who acted on their own[12] also left the I.M.S. in an anomalous position. The private insurance scheme was linked to the possibilities of withdrawal, and the unlikelihood and discouragement of the latter reduced enthusiasm for the former. It was hoped among some in the B.M.A. leadership that the limited member interest would save the Association from the responsibility of starting the insurance. However, the General Practitioners' Association's sponsoring of an insurance scheme, no doubt, influenced B.M.A. activity for prestige reasons, and the private practices group maintained strong pressure to fulfill the insurance commitment. The marketing of the insurance, with its evident small support, would have the advantage of satisfying some of the membership, and at the same time clearing the air for more realistic policies.

The functioning of the B.M.A. during 1965–66 did much to confirm Eckstein's observations about the first decade of the Health Service when he concluded:

Far from being involved in constant warfare with the Ministry it [the B.M.A.] is engaged in constant cooperation with it—a highly useful adjunct to the Ministry's machinery of administration which, had it not already existed, the Ministry would have had to invent.[13]

Certainly by the end of the negotiations there was evident some irritation with those in the profession who continued to look dourly upon all arrangements with the Health Service. As was commented in the *B.M.A. Journal:*

Never before in the history of medicine has the medical profession in Britain, or elsewhere, known such security as in the N.H.S. Never before have doctors as a whole been so well off. Never before have they made such a fuss about their conditions of work or of their nobility or of their self-sacrifice. And never before, perhaps, have they been in such a position to make their presence felt. Because as a result of the brilliance of medical scientists, who have usually been badly paid, those who apply the fruits of their brains are able to make twice, three, or four times as much.[14]

The transition in the medical profession's culture from a private to a social contract has been greatly influenced by its environment. Although aware of the limitations of the Health Service, the British public has consistently supported it and the general principle of an egalitarian approach to health. This mandate has been so clearly evident that even governments and ministers unsympathetic to the Service have feared the political consequences of attacking its structure. The encouragement of the private sector and the right of consumer choice have been approved by some parties and governments since 1948, but the field of private medical practice can look to no measure which has significantly favored its growth. In retrospect, perhaps the most liberal terms were those extended by Bevan at the beginning of the Service when he was anxious to obtain the widest backing of the profession.

The advocates of the expansion of private practice have pointed to the increasing affluence of large sections of society which makes possible individual planning and investment for health needs. Even if the assumption of affluence is accepted, it does not necessarily provide a rationale for the private market. For, as both major political parties have realized when in power, medical care is a scarce social resource, and the primary task is making adequate health services available for all. Only in the case of a surplus could the choices of individual consumers be met without detracting significantly from the needs of the whole. The economic capacity of the consumer is not the only or even the essential determinant. However, even under optimum circumstances the consequences for the less well-to-do and for medical practitioners of two systems of medicine might well raise doubts as to its advisability. The experience of doctors in the National Health Service and their reaction to the demands of public and private practice provide an important guide to the essential unity of health policy.

Notes

INTRODUCTION

1. See Harry Eckstein, *The English Health Service*, Cambridge: Harvard University Press, 1959; Almont Lindsey, *Socialized Medicine in England and Wales*, Chapel Hill: University of North Carolina Press, 1962; Brian Abel-Smith, *The Hospitals*, Cambridge: Harvard University Press, 1964; Rosemary Stevens, *Medical Practice in Modern England*, New Haven: Yale University Press, 1966.

CHAPTER 1

1. H. C. Debs., 422, April 1946, p. 43.
2. *Report of the Committee of Enquiry into the Cost of the National Health Service*, Cmnd. 9663, London: HMSO, 1956, p. 156.
3. *Ibid.*
4. Almont Lindsey, *Socialized Medicine in England and Wales*, Chapel Hill: University of North Carolina Press, 1962, p. 6.
5. *Ibid.*, p. 11.
6. *Ibid.*, pp. 8–9.
7. *Ibid.*, pp. 11–12.
8. A. T. Page, *Pennies for Health*, British Hospitals Contributory Schemes Association, 1949, p. 30.
9. Quoted in *ibid.*, p. 58.
10. Brian Abel-Smith, *The Hospitals*, Cambridge: Harvard University Press, 1964.
11. Page, *Pennies for Health*, pp. 11 ff.
12. *Ibid.*, p. 57.
13. Abel-Smith, *The Hospitals*, pp. 399–401.
14. *Ibid.*, pp. 392–97.
15. Lindsey, *Socialized Medicine in England and Wales*, p. 16.
16. Abel-Smith, *The Hospitals*, pp. 368–80.

17. *Report of the Committee of Enquiry* . . ., p. 157; Abel-Smith, *The Hospitals*, p. 380.

18. Sir Robert Platt, *Doctor and Patient*, The Nuffield Provincial Hospitals Trust, 1963, pp. 15–16.

19. Ministry of Health, *A National Health Service*, Cmnd. 6502, London: HMSO, 1944, p. 9.

20. Ministry of Health, *National Health Service Bill*, Cmnd. 6791, London: HMSO, 1946, p. 3.

21. Ann Cartwright, *Patients and Their Doctors*, London: Routledge and Kegan Paul, 1967, Table 2.

22. Ann Cartwright and Rosalind Marshall, "General Practice in 1963," *Medical Care* 3(2):71 (April–June 1965).

23. Stephen J. Hadfield, "A Field Survey of General Practice, 1951–2," *British Medical Journal*, September 26, 1953, p. 699. The survey of the Royal Commission on Doctors' and Dentists' Remuneration (Cmnd. 939, London: HMSO, 1960, paragraph 116) reported that private practice, in 1955–56, was the main activity of 10 percent of the N.H.S. practices and the secondary activity of 25 percent. However, no data are given about how many of these were older, semi-retired physicians with limited practices.

24. This estimate is based on the data in Brian Abel-Smith and Kathleen Gales, *British Doctors at Home and Abroad*, Occasional Papers on Social Administration, No. 8, London: G. Bell, 1954, Table 8, p. 31. It conforms to the unofficial estimates of the British Medical Association, which have varied between 575 and 625 from 1956 to 1958. (See *British Medical Journal, Supplement*, April 7, 1956, p. 140 and May 10, 1958, p. 240.) In December 1957 the Minister of Health set the number of solely private practitioners at approximately 600. (*British Medical Journal*, December 7, 1957, p. 1376.) Most estimates appear to be influenced by the B.M.A.'s statistics on doctors in private practice. However, apart from its accuracy, the B.M.A. list cannot be interpreted as containing only doctors outside the N.H.S. but rather those "solely or predominantly" in private practice. (*British Medical Journal, Supplement*, May 10, 1958, p. 240). This has caused some difficulty for those estimating the proportions of those mainly in private practice since there has been a tendency to increase the B.M.A. total by the number of physicians "predominantly," but not "solely" in private practice—a group already to some extent, at least, on the B.M.A. list. See, for example, D. S. Lees, "Private General Practice and the National Health Service," *The Sociological Review Monograph*, No. 5, University of Keele, 1962, pp. 33–34. The B.M.A. in February 1952, estimated that the total of those with wholly private practices and "restricted" N.H.S. lists would not be "less than 1,000."

(Royal Commission on Doctors' Dentists' Remuneration, *Minutes of Evidence*, 5–6, p. 249.)

25. Stephen Taylor, *Good General Practice*, Oxford: Oxford University Press, 1954, pp. 18–19. At that time, he estimated there were 450 private general practitioners or 2½ percent of the total.

26. *British Medical Journal*, December 5, 1965, p. 1555.

27. See *British Medical Journal*, February 27, 1965, p. 598, for practitioner income.

28. P. G. Gray and Ann Cartwright, "Choosing and Changing Doctors," *Lancet*, December 19, 1953, p. 1308.

29. Cartwright, *Patients and Their Doctors*, p. 8.

30. D. S. Lees, "Private General Practice and the National Health Service," pp. 35–36.

31. Abel-Smith and Gales, *British Doctors at Home and Abroad*, p. 34.

32. Fellowship for Freedom in Medicine, *Bulletin 26*, October 1954, pp. 12–14.

33. Paul F. Gemmill, *Britain's Search for Health*, Philadelphia: University of Pennsylvania Press, 1960, p. 84.

34. Royal Commission on Doctors' and Dentists' Remuneration, *Minutes of Evidence*, 5–6, p. 245.

35. Ministry of Health, *Annual Report, 1964*, Cmnd. 2688, London: HMSO, 1965, Table 62, p. 144.

36. Royal Commission on Doctors' and Dentists' Remuneration, *Minutes of Evidence*, 21, p. 1133.

37. *Ibid.*, p. 1135.

38. Royal Commission on Doctors' and Dentists' Remuneration, *Report, 1957–1960*, Cmnd. 939, London: HMSO, 1960, Table 18, p. 268.

39. *Ibid.*, Table 28, p. 79.

40. Royal Commission on Doctors' and Dentists' Remuneration, *Minutes of Evidence*, 21, p. 1134.

41. Ministry of Health, *Digest of Health Service Statistics*, 1963, Series A, No. 9, Statistics Branch, London: HMSO, 1964, Tables 1 and 2, p. 2.

42. Based on statistics in *The Hospitals Year Book, 1965*, London: The Institute of Hospital Administrators, 1965, pp. 450–69.

43. Lindsey, *Socialized Medicine in England and Wales*, p. 280.

44. Royal Commission on Doctors' and Dentists' Remuneration, *Minutes of Evidence*, 21, p. 1135.

45. E. F. Webb, "Independent Medical Practice," Fellowship for Freedom in Medicine, *Bulletin 57*, February 1964, p. 26.

CHAPTER 2

1. Royal Commission on Doctors' and Dentists' Remuneration, *Minutes of Evidence, 1*, p. 40; *Minutes of Evidence, 21*, p. 1135; *see also* the Fellowship for Freedom in Medicine *Bulletin.*

2. Brian Abel-Smith, *The Hospitals*, Cambridge: Harvard University Press, 1964, p. 499.

3. *Ibid.*, p. 465.

4. British Hospitals Contributory Schemes Association, *Second Annual Report*, 1949–1950, p. 4.

5. Sidney Lamb, "The Future Policy of Voluntary Hospital Contributory Schemes," address to Yorkshire Branch of Incorporated Association of Hospital Officers, April 19, 1941 (unpublished).

6. *Minutes* of the Conference of October 30, 1946, for discussion of the proposal to form a national provident association, p. 18 (unpublished).

7. *Report* of the Conference of October 30, 1946, for discussion of the proposal to form a national provident association (mimeographed).

8. The data on the societies' memberships and incomes are taken from the annual reports of the societies and supplemented by personal communications with executives of the societies. The statistics from the different societies are not entirely comparable due to differences in the financial years used by the societies.

9. See Fellowship for Freedom in Medicine, *Bulletin 41*, February 1959, pp. 22–23.

10. The British United Provident Association, *Sixteenth Annual Report*, June 30, 1963, p. 2.

11. *British Medical Journal, Supplement*, July 25, 1964, p. 54.

12. The British United Provident Association, *Tenth Annual Report*, June 30, 1957, p. 3.

13. *Ibid., Eighteenth Annual Report*, June 30, 1965, p. 7.

14. Ralph Harris and Michael Solly, *A Survey of Large Companies*, London: Institute of Economic Affairs, 1959, p. 22 and Table 19; G. L. Reid and James Bates, "The Cost of Fringe Benefits in British Industry," *Fringe Benefits, Labor Costs, and Social Security*, G. L. Reid and D. J. Robertson, eds., London: Allen & Unwin, 1965, pp. 73, 90.

15. The Hospital Service Plan, *Private Patients Plan*, p. 1.

16. *Ibid., Management and Staff Illness*, p. 1.

17. Ralph Harris and Arthur Seldon, *Choice in Welfare*, London: Institute of Economic Affairs, 1965.

18. British Hospitals Contributory Schemes Association, *Sixth Annual Report*, 1953.

19. *Ibid.*, *Seventeenth Annual Report*, 1965, p. 12.
20. John Dodd, "Supplementing Insurance" (n.d.; printed).
21. British Hospitals Contributory Schemes Association, *Seventeenth Annual Report*, 1965, p. 13.
22. *Ibid.*, *Fifteenth Annual Report*, 1963, p. 7.
23. Based on British Hospital Contributory Schemes Association, *Directory of Hospital Contributory Schemes Benefits*, 1964.
24. Based on statistics of The Hospital Saving Association, *Forty-third Annual Report*, 1965, p. 12.
25. British Hospitals Contributory Schemes Association, *Fifteenth Annual Report*, 1963, p. 7.
26. *Report of the Chief Registrar of Friendly Societies, 1964*, London: HMSO, 1965, Pt. 2, *Friendly Societies*, p. 17.
27. *Ibid.*, Table D, p. 30.
28. *Ibid.*, Table C, p. 29.
29. *Ibid.*, p. 18.
30. *Ibid.*, Pt. 4, *Trade Unions*, p. 12.

CHAPTER 3

1. P. G. Gray and Ann Cartright, "Choosing and Changing Doctors," *Lancet*, December 19, 1953, p. 1308.
2. Ann Cartright and Rosalind Marshall, "General Practice in 1963," *Medical Care* 3(2):71 (April–June 1965).
3. Ann Cartright, *Human Relations and Hospital Care*, London: Routledge and Kegan Paul, 1964, p. 199.
4. Ralph Harris and Arthur Seldon, *Choice in Welfare*, London: Institute of Economic Affairs, 1965, p. 36.
5. *Ibid.*, Table 7.
6. See Political and Economic Planning, *Family Needs and the Social Services*, London: Allen & Unwin, 1961, pp. 54–57; Brian Abel-Smith and R. M. Titmuss, *The Cost of the National Health Service*, Cambridge: Cambridge University Press, 1965, pp. 148–52.
7. Ann Cartright, *Patients and Their Doctors*, London: Routledge and Kegan Paul, 1967, p. 10.
8. Stephen Taylor, *Good General Practice*, Oxford: Oxford University Press, 1954, p. 70.
9. Harris and Seldon, *Choice in Welfare*, Table 7.
10. *British Medical Journal, Supplement*, July 17, 1965, 58.
11. Paul Ferris, *The Doctors*, London: Victor Gollancz, 1965, pp. 136–37.

12. For a dramatic description of surgery in a London nursing home, see Peter Mannigan, *Goodbye, Doctor, Goodbye*, London: Abelard-Schuman, 1963, pp. 72–75.
13. H. C. Debs., 422, May 1946, pp. 256–60.
14. Cartwright, *Patients and Their Doctors*, p. 11.
15. Taylor, *Good General Practice*, p. 72.

CHAPTER 4

1. H. C. Debs., 454, July 1948, p. 36.
2. *Ibid.*, 472, March 1950, p. 2136.
3. *British Medical Journal, Supplement*, September 8, 1956, p. 123.
4. Fellowship for Freedom in Medicine, "The Preservation of Private Practice," Broadsheet 7 (April 1956).
5. *British Medical Journal, Supplement*, July 1, 1961, p. 12; July 29, 1961, p. 93.
6. *Ibid.*, March 13, 1965, p. 93.
7. *Ibid.*, February 25, 1961, pp. 66–67
8. *Ibid.*, April 18, 1959, pp. 186.
9. Fellowship for Freedom in Medicine, "The Preservation of Private Practice."
10. *British Medical Journal, Supplement*, August 1, 1964, p. 81.
11. *Ibid.*, p. 80.
12. *Ibid.*, August 21, 1954, p. 99; Donald M. Johnson, *The British National Health Service*, London: Johnson, 1962, pp. 139–40.
13. Fellowship for Freedom in Medicine, *Bulletin 46*, January 1961, pp. 7, 13.
14. Quoted in *ibid.*, *Bulletin 43*, January 1960, p. 15.
15. *British Medical Journal, Supplement*, June 19, 1965, pp. 274–75.
16. H. C. Debs., 458, December 1948, p. 202.
17. *Ibid.*, 475, May 1950, p. 565.
18. *British Medical Journal, Supplement*, July 17, 1964, p. 40.
19. *British Medical Journal*, October 23, 1954, p. 975.
20. *British Medical Journal, Supplement*, April 7, 1956, p. 140.
21. Almont Lindsey, *Socialized Medicine in England and Wales*, Chapel Hill: University of North Carolina Press, 1962, p. 203.
22. Fellowship for Freedom in Medicine, "The Preservation of Private Practice"; *British Medical Journal, Supplement*, February 7, 1959, pp. 49–50.

23. H. C. Debs., 498, April 1952, p. 126; *British Medical Journal*, April 18, 1959, 1053; *British Medical Journal, Supplement*, June 19, 1965, 275.

24. *British Medical Journal, Supplement*, October 16, 1954, p. 145.

25. *British Medical Journal*, October 23, 1954, p. 975.

26. *Ibid.;* Fellowship for Freedom in Medicine, "The Preservation of Private Practice."

27. Fellowship for Freedom in Medicine, *Bulletin 46*, January 1961, p. 13, estimate of 36 percent agrees with estimates given author by other doctors and generally conforms to estimates used in establishing private practice insurance schemes.

28. *British Medical Journal*, May 13, 1965, p. 718.

29. See, for example, survey conducted by the Fellowship for Freedom in Medicine, *Bulletin 26*, October 1954, pp. 13–14; *A Review of the Medical Services in Great Britain* (The Porritt Committee Report) London: HMSO, 1962, p. 35.

30. See Gallup Poll survey reported in the Porritt Committee Report, p. 212; Political and Economic Planning, *Family Needs and the Social Services*, London: Allen & Unwin, 1961, p. 100.

31. *British Medical Journal, Supplement*, September 26, 1953, p. 114.

32. Ministry of Health, *National Health Service Bill*, Cmnd. 6761, London: HMSO, 1946, p. 10.

33. *Ibid.*, p. 8.

34. H. C. Debs., 422, April 1946, p. 57.

35. *British Medical Journal, Supplement*, July 23, 1949, pp. 53–54.

36. S. R. Speller, *Law Relating to Hospitals*, London: H. K. Lewis, 1965, p. 440.

37. *Ibid.*, p. 443.

38. *Annual Report* of the Ministry of Health, 1949, Cmnd. 7910, London: HMSO, 1950, p. 251.

39. *Ibid.*

40. *Ibid.*

41. Ministry of Health, *Digest of Health Service Statistics*, 1963, Series A, No. 9, Statistics Branch, London: HMSO, 1964, Tables 1 and 2, p. 2.

42. *British Medical Journal, Supplement*, February 29, 1964, p. 60.

43. *Ibid.*, February 22, 1964, p. 49.

44. Ministry of Health, *Digest of Health Service Statistics*, 1963, Table 2, p. 2.

45. *Ibid.*

46. *Ibid.*

47. *Ibid.*, Table 1, p. 2.

48. *British Medical Journal, Supplement,* December 19, 1964, p. 223.
49. D. S. Lees and M. H. Cooper, "Amenity and Private Pay-Beds," *British Medical Journal, Supplement,* June 8, 1963, pp. 1531–33.
50. *British Medical Journal, Supplement,* July 4, 1964.
51. *British Medical Journal,* May 15, 1954, p. 1161.
52. National Health Service, "Review of Pay Beds," H.M.(66) 26, April 1, 1966.
53. Lees and Cooper, "Amenity and Private Pay-Beds," p. 1533.
54. Letter from B.M.A. to author, November 9, 1965.
55. National Health Service, "The National Health Service (Pay-Bed Accommodation in Hospitals, etc.) Regulations, 1953," R.H.B. (53) 26 H.M.C. (53) 24 B.G. (53) 26, March 18, 1953, p. 420.
56. Royal Commission on Doctors' and Dentists' Remuneration, *Minutes of Evidence, 21,* p. 1095.
57. *British Medical Journal,* February 5, 1966, pp. 367–68.
58. Based on figures in *The Hospital Year Book,* 1951–1962, Secs. 8 and 9.
59. Letter from B.M.A. to author, November 9, 1965.
60. *A Review of the Medical Services in Great Britain,* paragraph 126; Royal Commission on Doctors' and Dentists' Remuneration, *Minutes of Evidence, 21,* p. 1095; *Report of the Committee of Enquiry into the Cost of the National Health Service* Cmnd. 9663, London: HMSO, 1956, paragraph 422.
61. See, for example, Royal Commission on Doctors' and Dentists' Remuneration, *Minutes of Evidence, 21,* p. 1095.
62. *British Medical Journal, Supplement,* July 20, 1963, pp. 35–36.
63. *Ibid.,* May 25, 1963, p. 246.
64. *Report of the Committee of Enquiry* . . . paragraph 423.
65. *Ibid.,* paragraph 420.
66. H. C. Debs., 422, May 1946, p. 218.
67. National Health Services, "The National Health Service (Pay-Bed Accommodation in Hospitals, etc.) Regulations, 1948," National Health Service, 1948, p. 1490.
68. *Ibid.,* paragraph 228.
69. *Ibid.,* paragraph 9.
70. *British Medical Journal, Supplement,* March 28, 1953, pp. 94–95; *British Medical Journal,* May 9, 1953, p. 1056.
71. *Ibid.*
72. National Health Service, "The National Health Service (Pay-Bed Accommodation in Hospitals, etc.) Regulations, 1953," R.H.B. (53) 26 H.M.C. (53) 24 B.G. (53) 26, March 18, 1953, p. 420.
73. BBC Script, "Panorama," November 22, 1965.

74. *Medical News,* August 20, 1965, p. 24.
75. E. F. Webb, "Independent Medical Practice," Fellowship for Freedom in Medicine, *Bulletin* 57, February 1964, p. 32.
76. National Health Service, "Signing of Undertakings by Private Patients," R.H.B. (53) 111 H.M.C. (53) 105 B.G. 107, November 12, 1953.
77. National Health Service, "The National Health Service (Pay-Bed Accommodation in Hospitals, etc.) Regulations, 1953," R.H.B. (53) 26 H.M.C. (53) 24 B.G. (53) 26, March 18, 1953, paragraph 15.
78. *Ibid.,* paragraph 16.
79. *Medical News,* August 20, 1965, p. 24.
80. Memorandum of the Central Consultants and Specialists Committee of B.M.A., *British Medical Journal, Supplement,* July 17, 1965, p. 71.
81. Letter from B.U.P.A. to author, May 11, 1966.
82. Letter from Hospital Service Plan to author, June 6, 1966.
83. *British Medical Journal,* February 5, 1966, pp. 367–68.
84. *Ibid.,* May 9, 1953, p. 1056.
85. *British Medical Journal, Supplement,* October 9, 1954, p. 1381.
86. Lindsey, *Socialized Medicine in England and Wales,* p. 277.
87. National Health Service, "Review of Pay-Beds," H.M.(66) 26, April 1, 1966, paragraph 4.
88. Lindsey, *Socialized Medicine in England and Wales,* p. 278.
89. *British Medical Journal, Supplement,* July 20, 1963, 35–36; July 4, 1964, 10–11.
90. *Report of the Committee of Enquiry . . . ,* paragraph 419.
91. See "Pertinax," *British Medical Journal,* May 28, 1966, 1355.
92. Lindsey, *Socialized Medicine in England and Wales,* p. 130.
93. Review Body on Doctors' and Dentists' Remuneration, *Fifth Report,* Cmnd. 2585, London: HMSO, 1965, p. 11.
94. Royal Commission on Doctors' and Dentists' Remuneration, *Report, 1957–1960,* Cmnd. 939, London: HMSO, 1960, paragraph 342.
95. Review Body on Doctors' and Dentists' Remuneration, *Seventh Report,* Cmnd. 2992, London: HMSO, 1966, paragraph 154.
96. B.M.A., "Family Doctor Service," *Second Report of Joint Discussions between General Practitioner Representatives and the Minister of Health,* 1965, paragraph 16.
97. Royal Commission on Doctors' and Dentists' Remuneration, *Minutes of Evidence, 3–4,* p. 147.
98. *Ibid.,* 9, p. 451.
99. *Ibid.,* pp. 451–55.

100. Royal Commission on Doctors' and Dentists' Remuneration, *Report, 1957–1960,* paragraph 331.

101. Review Body on Doctors' and Dentists' Remuneration, *Seventh Report,* paragraph 213.

102. *Doctor's Remuneration, The GPA Report,* Pt. 2, London: General Practitioners' Association, 1964, pp. 30–31.

103. Royal Commission on Doctors' and Dentists' Remuneration, *Report, 1957–1960,* p. 61.

104. Roger Ormrod and Harry Walker, *The National Health Service,* London: Butterworth, 1950, pp. 29–30.

105. Ministry of Health, *Report of the Inter-Departmental Committee on the Remuneration of Consultants and Specialists,* Cmnd. 7420, London: HMSO, 1948, paragraph 15.

106. *Ibid.*

107. Royal Commission on Doctors' and Dentists' Remuneration, *Report, 1957–1960,* paragraph 207–09.

108. *Ibid.,* paragraph 206.

109. Royal Commission on Doctors' and Dentists' Remuneration, *Written Evidence, 1,* London: HMSO, 1957, p. 19.

110. *Report of the Inter-Departmental Committee,* paragraph 12.

111. Royal Commission on Doctors' and Dentists' Remuneration, *Report, 1957–1960,* Table 28, p. 79; Table 25, pp. 76–77; see also Ministry of Health, *Annual Report, 1964,* Cmnd. 2688, London: HMSO, 1964, Table 71, pp. 164–65.

112. See Royal Commission on Doctors' and Dentists' Remuneration, *Minutes of Evidence,* 3–4.

113. Editorial, *Lancet,* July 15, 1961, pp. 148–49.

114. National Health Service, "Appointment of Consultants," HM (66) 14, February 25, 1966, Appendix.

115. Brian Abel-Smith and Richard M. Titmuss, *The Cost of the National Health Service,* Cambridge: Cambridge University Press, 1964, pp. 122–26.

116. *British Medical Journal, Supplement,* August 5, 1961, 108.

117. *Ibid.,* May 11, 1963, 178–90; June 1, 1963, 260.

118. National Health Service, "Appointment of Consultants," HM (66), 14, February 25, 1966.

119. Royal Commission on Doctors' and Dentists' Remuneration, *Written Evidence, 1,* paragraph 403.

120. See D. S. Lees, *Health Through Choice,* Hobart Paper 14, London: Institute of Economic Affairs, 1951.

121. R. S. Murley, "Alternative and Supplementary Systems of Financing Medical Care," Fellowship for Freedom in Medicine, *Bulletin 51,* August 1962, pp. 17–23.

122. See, for example, Fellowship for Freedom in Medicine, *Bulletin 34,* October 1956, pp. 6–7; *Bulletin 52,* October 1962, pp. 20–23.

123. *A Review of the Medical Services in Great Britain* (The Porritt Committee Report), London. HMSO, 1962, p. 36.

124. *British Medical Journal, Supplement,* March 27, 1954, 100.

125. *Ibid.,* July 10, 1954, 9.

126. Ralph Harris and Arthur Seldon, *Choice in Welfare,* London: Institute of Economic Affairs, 1965, Table 21.

127. *A Review of the Medical Services in Great Britain,* p. 233.

128. Harris and Seldon, *Choice in Welfare,* Table 8, p. 36.

129. *Ibid.,* p. 61.

CHAPTER 5

1. Ministry of Health, *Annual Report, 1964,* Cmnd. 2688, London: HMSO, 1965, Table 62, Pt. 1, p. 144.

2. Royal Commission on Doctors' and Dentists' Remuneration, *Report, 1957–1960,* Cmnd. 939, London: HMSO, 1960, Table 19, p. 62.

3. Brian Abel-Smith, *The Hospitals,* Cambridge: Harvard University Press, 1964, p. 473.

4. Stephen Taylor, *Good General Practice,* Oxford: Oxford University Press, 1954, p. 42.

5. Almont Lindsey, *Socialized Medicine in England and Wales,* Chapel Hill: University of North Carolina Press, 1962, p. 193.

6. Fellowship for Freedom in Medicine, *Bulletin 34,* October 1956, pp. 18–19.

7. See Ministry of Health, *Annual Report, 1964,* Table 61, Pt. 1, p. 134.

8. H. C. Debs., 425, July 1946, p. 1779.

9. *A Review of the Medical Services in Great Britain* (the Porritt Committee Report), London: HMSO, 1962, p. 34.

10. Lindsey, *Socialized Medicine in England and Wales,* p. 192.

11. Standing Medical Advisory Committee, Central Health Services Council, *The Field of Work of the Family Doctor,* London: HMSO, 1964, paragraph 164.

12. See Royal Commission on Doctors' and Dentists' Remuneration, *Minutes of Evidence, 3–4,* Cmnd. 936, London: HMSO, 1960; Lindsey, *Socialized Medicine in England and Wales,* pp. 191–92.

13. See Harry Eckstein, *The English Health Service,* Cambridge: Harvard University Press, 1959.

14. Royal Commission on Doctors' and Dentists' Remuneration, *Report, 1957–1960,* paragraph 331.

15. *British Medical Journal, Supplement,* May 22, 1954, 249; July 14, 1956, 16–17.

16. *Ibid.,* July 2, 1960, 26.

17. *Ibid.,* July 14, 1956, 16–17.

18. *Ibid.,* February 8, 1958, 52.

19. *Ibid., March* 13, 1965, 93.

20. Review Body on Doctors' and Dentists' Remuneration, *Seventh Report,* Cmnd. 2992, London: HMSO, 1966, paragraph 213.

21. *British Medical Journal, Supplement,* October 3, 1964, p. 142; June 19, 1965, p. 275.

22. Fellowship for Freedom in Medicine, *Bulletin* 37, November 1957, pp. 6–7.

23. Royal Commission on Doctors' and Dentists' Remuneration, *Minutes of Evidence,* 21, p. 1091.

24. *Ibid.*

25. *Ibid.,* p. 1096.

26. *Ibid.,* 1, p. 38–39.

27. L. L. W. Peters, "Hewers of Wood and Drawers of Water," *Lancet,* September 19, 1964, pp. 634–37.

28. *Report of the Committee of Enquiry into the Cost of the National Health Service,* Cmd. 9663, London: HMSO, 1956, paragraph 400.

29. H. C. Debs., 452, June 1948, p. 1551.

30. *British Medical Journal, Supplement,* January 3, 1959, p. 4.

31. *Ibid.,* October 16, 1954, p. 145.

32. *Ibid.,* April 29, 1961; Letter to editor, *Lancet,* April 1, 1961, pp. 718–19.

33. *British Medical Journal, Supplement,* July 17, 1965, 58.

34. H. C. Debs., 723, January 1966, p. 680.

35. Ann Cartwright, *Human Relations and Hospital Care,* London: Routledge and Kegan Paul, 1964, pp. 27–28.

36. *Ibid.*

37. Robert Hewer, "The Widdecombe File," *Lancet,* January 14, 1961, p. 91.

38. H. C. Debs., 452, June 1948, pp. 1548–51.

39. Lindsey, *Socialized Medicine in England and Wales,* p. 59.

40. See Eckstein, *The English Health Service,* pp. 154–55 for a discussion of medical "politicians."

41. See D. S. Lees, "Private General Practice and the National

Health Service," *Sociological Review Monograph*, No. 5, University of Keele, 1962, pp. 38–39.

42. Ann Cartwright and Rosalind Marshall, "General Practice in 1963," *Medical Care*, 3(2):71 (April–June 1965).

43. *Ibid.*

44. *British Medical Journal, Supplement*, February 7, 1959, p. 49.

45. Cartwright and Marshall, "General Practice in 1963," p. 72.

46. *Ibid.*, p. 71.

47. Royal Commission on Doctors' and Dentists' Remuneration, *Minutes of Evidence*, 21, paragraph 5121.

48. Joseph S. Collings, "General Practice in England Today," *Lancet*, March 25, 1950, p. 569.

49. *British Medical Journal, Supplement*, September 11, 1954, p. 116.

50. Cartwright and Marshall, "General Practice in 1963," p. 72.

51. *British Medical Journal, Supplement*, July 17, 1965, p. 67.

52. *A Review of the Medical Services in Great Britain*, p. 41.

53. Ministry of Health, "Helping Your Doctor," 1965.

54. Stephen J. Hadfield, "A Field Survey of General Practice, 1951–2," *British Medical Journal*, September 26, 1953, p. 670.

55. W. I. D. Scott, "Ethics of Private Practice with an N.H.S., *Medical World Newsletter*, November 1965, pp. 22–23.

56. *British Medical Journal, Supplement*, September 26, 1953, p. 113.

57. *Ibid.*

58. Royal Commission on Doctors' and Dentists' Remuneration, *Minutes of Evidence*, 3–4, p. 108.

59. *British Medical Journal, Supplement*, October 14, 1950, p. 653.

60. Lindsey, *Socialized Medicine in England and Wales*, pp. 142–48.

61. *British Medical Journal*, July 3, 1965, p. 55; May 8, 1965, p. 1252.

62. Lindsey, *Socialized Medicine in England and Wales*, p. 147.

63. R. Hale-White, "Stop Looking Backward," Fellowship for Freedom in Medicine, *Bulletin 63*, February 1966, p. 33.

64. Fellowship for Freedom in Medicine, *Bulletin 61*, June 1965, p. 12.

65. *Ibid.*, p. 10.

66. Fellowship for Freedom in Medicine, *Bulletin 62*, November 1965, p. 25.

67. *Medical World Newsletter*, April 1965, p. 3.

68. All the following references to the Charter are found in the

publication of the British Medical Association, *A Charter for the Family Doctor Service,* March 8, 1965.

69. "Family Doctor Service, *Second Report of Joint Discussions between General Practitioner Representatives and the Minister of Health,*" London: B.M.A., 1965, Appendix D.

70. *British Medical Journal, Supplement,* April 3, 1965, p. 123.

71. *British Medical Journal,* November 6, 1965, p. 1076.

72. _____. "Health and Social Class," *Lancet,* April 3, 1965, pp. 745–46.

73. *British Medical Journal, Supplement,* July 3, 1965, p. 1.

74. *British Medical Journal,* February 27, 1965, p. 576.

75. *British Medical Journal, Supplement,* October 21, 1950, p. 170.

76. *British Medical Journal,* January 15, 1966, p. 171.

77. *British Medical Journal, Supplement,* October 23, 1965, p. 177.

78. *Ibid.,* July 17, 1965, p. 42.

79. *Ibid.,* December 18, 1965, p. 244; October 30, 1965, 180.

80. *Ibid.,* April 30, 1966, p. 114.

81. *Ibid.,* December 18, 1965, p. 244.

82. *Ibid.,* April 2, 1966, p. 89; April 30, 1966, 114.

83. *Ibid.,* July 17, 1965, p. 42.

84. *Ibid.,* December, 18, 1965, p. 244.

85. *Ibid.,* April 30, 1966, p. 115.

86. *Ibid.,* May 7, 1966, p. 145.

87. *Ibid.,* April 30, 1966, p. 114.

88. Independent Medical Services, *Doctor's Booklet,* June 1966.

89. *Ibid.*

90. *Ibid.*

91. *British Medical Journal, Supplement,* September 11, 1965, p. 129.

92. *Ibid.,* April 30, 1966, p. 114.

93. *The Times,* July 2, 1966, p. 11.

94. *The Observer,* May 1, 1966, p. 1.

95. General Practitioners' Association, *The Family Care Service,* 1966.

96. Independent Medical Services, *Doctors' Booklet.*

97. General Practitioners' Association, *The Family Care Service,* 1966.

98. *British Medical Journal, Supplement,* August 21, 1965, p. 121.

99. *British Medical Journal,* August 14, 1965, p. 229.

100. *Ibid.,* January 1, 1966, p. 57.

101. *Medical Tribune,* April 28, 1966, p. 7.

102. *Ibid.*

103. Anne Lapping, "Birmingham's N.H.S. Rebellion," *New Soci-*

ety, August 19, 1965, pp. 18–19.

104. *British Medical Journal, Supplement,* July 10, 1965, p. 27.

105. Lapping, "Birmingham's N.H.S. Rebellion," p. 18.

106. *Ibid.,* p. 19.

CHAPTER 6

1. See Brian Abel-Smith and Kathleen Gales, *British Doctors at Home and Abroad,* Occasional Papers on Social Administration, No. 8, London: G. Bell, 1964.

2. *British Medical Journal, Supplement,* June 1, 1963, p. 260.

3. Sir Robert Platt, *Doctor and Patient,* The Nuffield Provincial Hospitals Trust, p. 18.

4. Robert Hewer, "The Widdecombe File," *Lancet,* January 14, 1961, p. 105.

5. See Ann Cartwright, *Patients and Their Doctors,* London: Routledge and Kegan Paul, 1967, Chap. IV.

6. See Standing Medical Advisory Committee, Central Health Services Council, *The Field of Work of the Family Doctors,* London: HMSO, 1963, particularly Sec. XVI.

7. Rosemary Stevens, *Medical Practice in Modern England,* New Haven: Yale University Press, 1966, pp. 359–61.

8. *British Medical Journal, Supplement,* February 6, 1965, p. 40; July 17, 1965, p. 67; November 20, 1965; pp. 212–13.

9. *Ibid.,* January 30, 1965.

10. *British Medical Journal,* February 27, 1965, p. 598.

11. *British Medical Journal, Supplement,* June 19, 1965, pp. 264–65.

12. *British Medical Journal,* August 14, 1965, p. 382.

13. Harry Eckstein, *Pressure Group Politics,* London: Allen & Unwin, 1960, p. 48.

14. "Pertinax," *British Medical Journal,* June 4, 1966, p. 1417.

Index

Abbreviations Used:
B.M.A.   British Medical Association
B.U.P.A. British United Provident Association
I.M.S.   Independent Medical Services
N.H.S.   National Health Service

"Amenity" beds: privacy provided by, 7; use of, 49

Bevan, Aneurin: approval of joint private and public health service, 34–35, 75; on availability of drugs for private patients, 38; defense of pay-bed use by private patients, 44–52; response to criticism, 77
Birmingham Action Group, 73: opposition to two types practice, 83; group resignation by, 85–86; question of free drugs, 94; and independent practice, 95–97; declining interest in, 100
Bow Group, 24–25
British Hospitals Contributory Schemes Association, 2–3, 28
British Medical Association: approval of capitation system of payment, 5; list of unreliable practitioners, 7–8; decline in private practice, 10; health insurance plan for doctors, 17; statement of issues in private practice, 37; question of free drugs, 38–39, 40–41, 42, 43, 71, 94; pressure for increase of private beds, 45, 46; estimate of cost of pay-beds, 48; approval of Review Body proposals, 55; threat of mass resignation

from N.H.S., 57; scheme of insurance for private practice, 57; review of opting out of N.H.S., 66; list of private practitioners criticized, 72; and fee-for-service proposal, 80, 86; and two types of practice, 83; formation of Medical Guild, 83–84; and the "Doctors' Strike," 85; internal struggle, 86; Charter, 86–88, 101, 102; insurance scheme, 89–91; salary system, 101; future role, 102
British Medical Guild, 83–84
British Medical Journal: on question of drugs to private patients, 39; on doctors' resignations, 88; on conditions in 1965, 103–04
British United Provident Association, 12–13; connection with private practice, 14–15; amalgamation with local associations, 16; domination of, 16; question of inclusion of drugs, 17–18; costs met by, 18; scheme for additional benefits, 18; in-patient benefits, 18; private charges paid, 18–19; maximum yearly grant extended, 19; scale of benefits, 20; age structure of subscribers, 21–22; rebates allowed, 22; Company sponsorship of hospital plans,

22–23; group management of insurance, 23; proportion of income spent on claims, 23; reserve position, 23; expenditures for development, 24; publicity, 24; and choice, 25; rates compared to contributory societies, 28; and abuses of fee system, 50; and abolition of fee system, 51

Carling, Sir Ernest Rock, 16
Central Consultants Committee: criticism by, 46; negotiations, 53
Cohen Committee, 41
Cohen, Sir Henry, 43
Conservative party: and Bow Group, 25; criticism of, 40; on private practice, 53
Consultants: choices open to, 6–7; use of N.H.S. hospitals, 10–11, 59; average income, 11–12; awards, 12, 61–62; and fee schedule, 50; fees for use of facilities, 59–60; compensations from N.H.S., 60, 73; advantages, 60–61, 69, 70–71; income tax, 62; whole-time or part-time choice, 62–63, 69; decline of part-time service, 63, 99; freedom, 69; disadvantages, 73–74; financial inequalities removed, 74
Contributory societies: membership in 1948, 15; identification with working classes, 15–16, 26, 31; financial benefits, 16, 26; problems, 19; growth, 26; need for new types of benefits, 26–27; size of, 27–28; internal conflict, 28; new schemes, 28; rates, 28; future, 29

"Doctors' Strike," 85–89

Eckstein, Harry, 103

Family Care Service, 94
Fellowship for Freedom in Medicine, 10, 37; and drugs for private patients, 40; suggested savings in drugs, 42; and drug scheme, 43; and cost of pay-beds, 48; opponent of N.H.S., 65, 98; and private health insurance, 65; criticism of B.M.A., 72–73; on mass resignations, 84–85
Financial Times, 25
Friendly societies: role in health insurance, 29; service after adoption of N.H.S., 29

Gallup Poll, 88
Gemmill, Paul, 10
General Medical Council, 38
General Medical Service Committee: on drug proposal, 71–72; and full-time requirement for general practitioners, 87
General practitioners: choices, 6; and private patients, 8; proportion of income from private and public service, 8–9; capitation fees, 54–55; acceptance of N.H.S., 54; patient list, 57; reliance on panel patients, 69; relationship with consultants, 69–70; use of hospitals, 70; morale, 70; and N.H.S. standards, 78; record keeping, 82–83; fee-for-service proposal, 83; remuneration, 83, 101; mass resignations, 83–85, 87; proposals in B.M.A. Charter, 87; and B.M.A. insurance plan, 90–91, 93; and I.M.S., 92–93; Family Care Service, 94; and Birmingham doctors, 95–97; decline of attachment to private practice, 98–99; emigration, 98–99; role in total health system, 101
General Practitioners' Association, 85
Group Management Ltd., 23
Guillebaud Committee, 48, 49: on use of private beds, 53–54; and junior staff, 74; on "queue jumping," 76

Hospital and Specialist Services, 59
Hospital facilities, 10
Hospital Saturday Fund, 28
Hospital Savings Association, 3, 15, 27–28
Hospital Service Plan: proportion of income spent on claims, 23; expenditures for development, 24; abuses of fee system, 50
Hospitals and clinics, 7

Independent Medical Services Ltd., 91–92
—scheme: fee-for-service, 81; B.M.A.'s alternative, 84, 85; function, 86; progress, 89; response to, 90–91, 93; details of, 92–93; free drugs in, 94; decline of interest in, 100; position of, 103
Institute of Economic Affairs: publication of *Choice in Welfare*, 24; on provident and contributory insurance, 31; survey on question of opting out of N.H.S., 66

Joint Consultants Committee, 11, 12, 44, 45, 49, 73
Jones, Dr. Ivor, chairman of Private Practices Committee of the B.M.A.: 89; support of insurance scheme, 91

Labour government: support of selective privilege of patients, 6; indifference to private practice, 102
Lancet: criticism of operation of Health Service, 76; summary of problems of private practice, 99
League of Hospital Friends, 26
Lees and Cooper survey, 46
Local Medical Committees, 88
London Association for Hospital Services, 16, 17; scheme of benefit payments, 18; changes in financial schemes, 19; surcharge for older subscribers, 22

Medical Practice Freedom Fund, 96
Medical Practitioners' Union, 85

Ministers of Health (Conservative and Labour parties), 8, 15, 41–42; and problems of hospitalization, 33, 44–49; opposition to private practice, 41; opposition to free drug scheme, 43, 71; concern with occupancy of hospital beds, 44–49; surveillance of specialists' charges, 50–51; proposed abandonment of fee system, 52; and part-time option, 63; criticism of N.H.S., 76; and the "Doctors' Strike," 88

National Health Service: act creating, xi, xii, 1, 5; early features of, 5–6; conception of by Conservative and Labour governments, 6; mixed practice, 6; types of hospital accommodation, 7; statistics of private practice under, 8; enrollment, 8–9; decline of private practice under, 10, 37; private beds, 10, 13, 21, 45–46; patients' choices, 13; growth of provident societies, 17, 25; home care provided, 18; limitations of, 25; charges for dentures and glasses, 26; criticism of, 34, 100–01; consideration of patients, 35; on question of drugs for private patients, 39; satisfaction with, 43, 104; cost schedules compared to private beds, 48; fees for private practice, 49–50; system of divided practice under, 54–55; Review Body's recommendations, 55; question of opting out, 66–67; shortcomings, 75; competence of doctors, 75; rumors about, 76; medical standards, 78–79; patient relations, 81; professional rights, 81; benefits from private patient plan, 81–82; simplification of private practice plan, 82; resignation of doctors, 84–85; "Doctors' Strike," 89; I.M.S. scheme proposed to, 92–93; effect of Bir-

mingham doctors' revolt, 95–97;
voluntary membership, 100; prob-
able evolution of, 101
National Health Insurance Scheme:
early coverage under, 1; benefits, 2
Nuffield, Lord, 16
Nuffield Nursing Home Trust, 12;
relations with B.U.P.A., 21, 23;
local contributions to, 21; publicity, 24; effort to increase private accommodation in public
hospitals, 46
Nursing homes: exemption from
nationalization, 12; demands on,
12; increase of, 12–13; limitations
of, 13

Panel system, 5
Pay-beds: increase of in 1930's, 4;
as source of income for private
practitioners, 7, 44; provision for
in public hospitals, 10, 44; in voluntary hospitals and nursing
homes, 12; rising costs of, 18, 21;
issue of increase of, 45–46; reduction of, 45; occupancy rate, 46;
variation in costs of, 47–48;
charges for, 49; use of, 52; restriction in use of, 53
"Penny a week" schemes, 27
Pilkington Commission, 55; effects
of joint service of doctors, 56–57;
question of private earnings in
pool practice, 58, 71; recommen-
dation for maintenance of part-
time service, 64; report on N.H.S.
care vs. private care, 79
Platt, Sir Robert: on early health
service, 5–6; on decline of interest
in private practice, 99
Poor Law, 4–5
Porritt Committee, 48; on tax allowances for private schemes, 65;
on opting out of N.H.S., 66
Provident Societies: coverage by in
1930's, 3, 5; coverage by in 1963,
13, 14; crisis, 15; identification
with upper classes, 16, 31; on in-

surance for private hospital care,
16; recruitment devices, 22; publicity and marketing functions,
23–24; advantages claimed by, 24;
position on issue of choice, 25;
growth of, 25, 26, 48–49; fee
schedule, 51–52; effect on private
practice, 68
Private practice: privileges under
N.H.S., 6, 64; role of, 9; class
range of, 30, 31; income as factor
in, 30, 31; continuation in "county
families," 30; and older patients,
31; ideology and custom as influence on, 32; appointment availability for, 32, 79; hospital availability for, 32–33; choice of
consultant, 33; use of private and
public services by, 33–34, 44; supply of drugs, 34, 38; social status
as motivation for use, 34–35, 78;
relation with doctor, 35, 80; privacy in hospitals, 36; criticism of
continued drug agitation, 39–40,
71, 72; problem of control of
drugs, 41, 43; provision for in
public hospitals, 44, 45, 70; laboratory and out-patient facilities
available to, 64; tax relief, 65; tax
subsidy, 66; three components of,
68; public tolerance, governmental indifference, support by doctors in growth of, 68; sources of
income for, 70; and recognition by
B.M.A., 71, 72; use of inadequacies of N.H.S., 76; more service
demanded by, 80; difference of attitude of doctor, 80–81; benefit to
the doctor of availability of public
care, 82; Birmingham doctors' effort to establish, 95–97; decline
of interest in, 99–101; support by
B.M.A., 102
Private Practices Committee: effort
to add drugs to B.U.P.A. scheme,
17–18, 39, 71–72; negotiations for
private hospital practice, 53; criticism by private practitioners, 72;

in "Doctors' Strike," 89; insurance scheme, 90; political influence, 102

Regional Hospital Boards, 45
Review Body: recommendations by, 55, 58; effect on income, 72
Royal Commission on Doctors' and Dentists' Remuneration, 11, 48

Specialists. *See* Consultants

Spens Committee: recommendations, 60; awards, 61
Western Provident Association, 16, 17; additional benefits paid by, 18; proportion of income spent on claims, 23; report on overcharges, 50; variations in charges, 51
White Paper of the Conservative government, 6
Whole-time Consultants' Association, 73